THE COMPLETE BOOK OF
SWEDISH
MASSAGE

THE COMPLETE BOOK OF

SWEDISH MASSAGE

BASED ON TECHNIQUES DEVELOPED BY PER HENRIK LING, M.D.

Armand Maanum
with Herb Montgomery

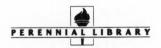

PERENNIAL LIBRARY

Harper & Row, Publishers, New York
Cambridge, Philadelphia, San Francisco, Washington
London, Mexico City, São Paulo, Singapore, Sydney

A paperback edition of this book
was originally published in 1985 by Winston Press, Inc.

THE COMPLETE BOOK OF SWEDISH MASSAGE. Copyright © 1985 by Armand Maanum with Herb Montgomery. All rights reserved. Printed in the United States of America. No part of this book may be used or reproduced in any manner whatsoever without written permission except in the case of brief quotations embodied in critical articles and reviews. For information address Harper & Row, Publishers, Inc., 10 East 53rd Street, New York, N.Y. 10022. Published simultaneously in Canada by Fitzhenry & Whiteside Limited, Toronto.

First PERENNIAL LIBRARY edition published in 1988.

Library of Congress Cataloging-in-Publication Data

Maanum, Armand.
   The complete book of Swedish massage.

   Bibliography: p.
   1. Massage.   2. Health.   I. Ling, Per Henrik, 1776–1839.   II. Montgomery, Herb.
III. Title.   IV. Title: Swedish massage.
RA780.5.M32   1988   615.8′22   87-45643
ISBN 0-06-097139-8 (pbk.)

88   89   90   91   92   MPC   10   9   8   7   6   5   4   3   2   1

CONTENTS

PART·ONE

The Gift of Touch   1

The Father of Swedish Massage   3
Massage and What It Can Do   8
Why Touch?   12
Sensitivity to Touch   15
Fear of Touch   18
Touch Misused   21
Sex and Massage   24
Can the Hands Heal?   28
Giving the Gift of Massage   31
Massage and Exercise   34

PART·TWO

Preparing for Massage   39

PART·THREE

Basic Hand Positions and Strokes   51

P A R T · F O U R

The Full Body Swedish Massage   69

The Feet   71
The Front of the Legs   79
The Abdomen   87
The Chest   91
The Hands   97
The Arms   105
The Back of the Neck   110
The Face   114
The Back of the Legs   124
The Lower Back   130
The Upper Back and Shoulders   135
The Deep Shoulder Blade   141
The Scalp   146
Wake Up Massage   150
Massage to Improve Regularity   152
Morning Massage   156
Eye Exercise and Massage   158
Relief for Leg Cramps   160
Relief for Joint Problems   162
Relief for Sinus, Tension, and Some Migraine
Headaches   164
Pregnancy Massage   166

Notes   169

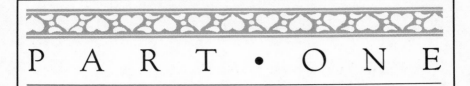

PART • ONE

The Gift of Touch

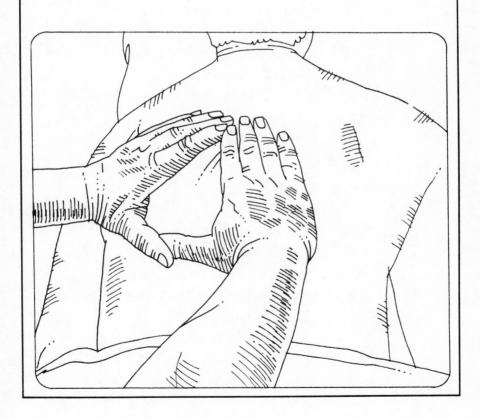

The Father
of Swedish Massage

Among the skills Scandinavian immigrants brought to America was Swedish massage. The art flourished wherever the immigrants settled, and it has been passed on from master to apprentice ever since. Although the basic elements of this massage have remained the same through the generations, its originator is seldom given the credit he deserves. Per (Peter) Henrik Ling was born in Sweden in 1776, the year Americans signed the Declaration of Independence. He was what we might refer to today as a renaissance man. Along with being a doctor and educator, he was a people's advocate and poet too.

Ling was well known in Sweden as a man who wrote both his poetry and other works in an impassioned and difficult-to-follow style. He believed in a poetry that would soothe the mind and bring good feelings. This interest in calming the mind with words sparked

Ling's interest in soothing the physical body as well. The year he turned twenty-nine, Ling took up fencing in order to learn more about its skillful movements. His study with two Frenchmen set down the framework of what would eventually become his *Svenska Gymnastikens* (Swedish exercise) system. Ling, in fact, is known as the father of Swedish exercising systems, which include his *Sjuk Gymnastikens Passiva Rorelser* (passive motion exercises of the sick, Ling's own name for Swedish massage). For this, he drew on all the knowledge he had acquired concerning health and physical activity and from his study of massage theories developed during the Greco-Roman days of games and contests. Of course he was also aware of the Nordic concepts of physical fitness in vogue during his lifetime. Eventually, he gathered what he considered the best of these ideas and formed a new system that was based on body physiology (functions of body organs) and body motion (exercises). He incorporated a third, and innovative, element—the conscious directing of the healing process by the mind towards the specific area of the body needing improvement.

Ling had a crusader's interest in teaching his new ideas to all the Swedish people, not just those of the aristocracy. He was particularly concerned that women and children be involved in physical fitness, including gymnastics. He was also concerned about applying his ideas to the needs of the military. To this end, he devised exercise routines that could be done with swords or other weapons in order to develop grace and balance. "Exercises with a purpose" might well be considered Ling's motto. His concern for combining beauty and motion led him to create a system of dance exercises to be performed to music. In a sense, he anticipated aerobic dancing, but his routines were somewhat less energetic, leaning more to the classical ballet style of dance.

Today's Swedish-style massages are the derivatives of Ling's original routines and many of the currently accepted techniques can be traced most directly to his medical concerns. The *Sjuk Gymnastikens Passiva Rorelser*, Ling's specially designed routines, have been somewhat diluted by the practitioners who followed him. Esalen-style massage is one of these derivatives. Ling was not particularly happy with the word "massage" because he considered it too general. If he'd had his way, we would know Swedish massage as "The Passive Motions of Medical Treatment of the Sick." Perhaps that would be a more precise term, but hardly memorable!

There is no doubt that Ling had a deeply inquisitive mind that led him to investigate a wide variety of interests. He took up the study of medicine and anatomy to assist him in developing his various exercise systems. He became a professor of medicine in 1825 and was named a professor of the Swedish Medical Society in 1831. His highest academic honor came in 1835, when he was named to the Swedish Royal Academy.

Today we would surely think of Ling as an activist. Certainly in the early 1800s his ideas were progressive, if not downright threatening to the ruling classes. He spoke out for common people's rights and was particularly concerned about the rights of women and female children. Ling not only founded schools but insisted that ordinary people had as much right to knowledge as did the rich and the aristocratic. Equally important, he insisted that people be taught to care for their bodies. Children did not play a secondary role in his thinking. In fact, Ling advocated that *all* children be exposed to exercise and the importance of maintaining their bodies. Although he may not have used the term, "wellness" was a central theme in Ling's lifelong work.

As word of Ling's ideas spread to other countries, his theories were ridiculed at first as bordering on the mystical or as the over-writing of a zealot, although "visionary" might have been a more apt description. Ling probably was too intense in his beliefs, but this is true of many innovators. We now know that Ling's systems are not always the cure-alls he envisioned them to be. They are, however, extremely helpful and do, in many cases, live up to his claims. For example, nerve blocks (the sending of false or no sensation to the brain) removed by massage techniques he designed often bring relief from pain and enable the body to heal itself.

In Ling's writings, we see that he also believed in treating the circulatory system and improving the posture, which he considered crucial to body health. How perceptive he was is demonstrated by the recognition by our current medical profession of the importance of good posture.

Ling lived a full and robust life of more than sixty years before dying in May of 1839. It wasn't until the 1900s, however, that his ideas began to be recognized and accepted around the world. Ling's son, Hjalmar, had carried on the teachings, but it was an English doctor named Roth who really became Ling's disciple and champion. Roth wrote books on Ling's original methods and may be credited with changing the thinking of his critics. What we now see in the life of Per Henrik Ling is a creative mind at work on a broad range of topics. From some of his research he devised new techniques to apply to body movement, exercise, and massage, using the empirical method. What worked, he incorporated; what didn't, he discarded. Thanks to this man's genius, the art of Swedish massage remains available today to anyone who is interested or in need of it.[1]

"'Exercise with a purpose' might well be considered Ling's motto."

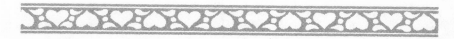

Massage
and What It Can Do

Massage is a controlled form of touching meant to create a particular response. Although the simpler forms can be learned by anyone, skilled practitioners spend a lifetime learning to read the body with fingers as sensitive and expertly trained as those required to read Braille. Massage is one of the most ancient of the healing arts and has many benefits, some of which can be easily measured. A simple hand massage stimulates the flow of blood to the hand and thus increases the skin temperature. Stimulating blood flow—which increases the delivery of nutrients as well as the elimination of wastes—is a basic benefit of all forms of massage. Tension-related headaches can be dispelled and others usually eased. Besides creating an overall sense of well-being, massage offers still other benefits. It can reduce swelling, relax muscles, relieve constipation.

Among the various types of massage currently popular in the United States are: *Shiatsu*, which is an Oriental massage involving the application of pressure through the balls of the thumbs; *Rolfing*, which can be severely painful, is a deep form of massage meant to reshape the body's posture; *Esalen* style, which is an outgrowth of the traditional European or Swedish massage. The specific massages presented later in this book are based on the original *Sjuk Gymnastikens Passiva Rorelser*, which I practice.

Swedish massage is an old and honorable healing art that was brought to the United States from Europe more than 100 years ago. Peter Henrik Ling combined what he considered to be the best techniques of the German, Italian, and other massage experts. Ling made two key contributions to the art by (1) devising motions that didn't require great strength and (2) standardizing a routine that could be taught to anyone, thus allowing a person to make a profession of massage.

The positive value of massage is recorded as long as 5,000 years ago, when Chinese physicians used it as a treatment for paralysis and other ailments. Today massage is a tool respected and used by nurses, physical therapists, chiropractors, and osteopaths. More and more, medical personnel are taking a renewed interest in the use of the hands for healing. Jules Older, a psychologist who writes and speaks about touching and healing, presents a convincing case for medical schools to include touch education, a subject that has been largely overlooked in the past. Of his own experience with massage Older says:

> What I have found is a deep relaxation . . . and a
> most soothing form of contact with another person. I

have received welcome relief for stiff and spasming muscles. And I have welcomed the gift of human comfort as my wife's fingers lift the veil of a dark mood from my eyes.

On the giving end, I have been able to use massage effectively to relieve cramps of the uterus and of the stomach, to loosen knotted muscles, and to relax a tense body.[2]

Dolores is a woman who has lived with intractable pain for many years. An auto accident and three back operations left her physically weak and susceptible to the debilitating pain that often results from fatigue as well as from sudden physical movements and rapid changes in the weather. Surgery, drugs, heat, cold, and traction were all forms of treatment she had experienced, but she had never considered massage. When we suggested she try it, Dolores was not only reluctant but skeptical. Finally she gave herself "permission" to go for a Swedish massage. What she found was not a cure, of course, but the results were immediate and beneficial. Massage helped loosen shoulder muscles she had unconsciously held in tension in an attempt to fight neck pain. Following her first massage, she moved more freely and enjoyed a second and unexpected benefit—a feeling of far more energy than she had been used to.

When we speak of the healing aspect of massage, we speak of healing in its broadest sense, of "bringing comfort." Dolores discovered that massage also put her actively in touch with her own body, and that it enabled her to be more caring in a personal relationship. She and her mother had a long history of being so uncomfortable in the presence of one another that they actually avoided contact. After a series of massages, Dolores discovered she was more sensitive not only to her own feelings but to those of others as well. She recognized the hurt in her mother and was surprised by what happened when the two of them went for a walk together. "I put my arm around her as we walked," Dolores said. "We talked and she cried and I cried and it was like a homecoming, a moment of healing."

"Massage is one of the most ancient of the healing arts and has many benefits, some of which can be easily measured."

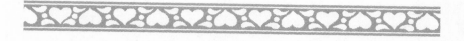

Why Touch?

Before giving the gift of massage to anyone, we should have a basic understanding of touch and its importance. It's believed that appropriate and compassionate touch is a critical factor in normal development for all of us and that it enhances physical, intellectual, and emotional growth.

Touching is a form of nourishment babies must have if they are to be healthy, and the need for tactile stimulation is lifelong. "To touch is far more than to soothe and massage the body physically," maintains Gay Luce who has worked extensively with the aged. Luce says, "[Touch] is the kind of nourishment that mothers give their infants, that lovers give each other, and that most adults give to cats and dogs—but not to each other."[3]

Anger is sometimes directed at people who focus more of their touch attention on pets and plants than on people. Recently studies have shown, however, that touching and caring for pets satisfies certain basic needs and may even extend life. Pets become a part of therapy. The elderly person who is confined to a wheelchair but has accepted the responsibility for a kitten will stroke and brush that animal and almost certainly grow to delight in doing so. It is the same with children. Those who must undergo long-term medical treatment appear happier when they can handle an animal that responds to their touch. There are even different animals for different temperaments: cats for the independent, snakes for the unconventional.

"Skin hunger" is the term that describes our need for touch. We may agree that touching is nourishment that satisfies our skin hunger, but do we all need it to survive? Is it really *that* important? Frederick Leboyer, a French obstetrician and gynecologist, says, "Being touched and caressed, being massaged, is food for the infant. Food as necessary as minerals, vitamins, and proteins. Deprived of this food, the name of which is love, babies would rather die. And they often do."[4] A Bellevue Hospital experience confirms the theory that physical contact with people increases a person's desire to live. When it was made hospital policy that children were to be given specific attention—to be picked up, held, and moved about on a daily basis—the rate of death changed. In one year, the incidence of child death decreased from over thirty percent to under ten percent.[5]

Truly, to touch is to give life. Many studies have indicated that people who are deprived of loving, caring touch deteriorate mentally and suffer in other ways as well. In a foundling home, young children who were otherwise cared for but went without the touch of other people were slow to speak, walk, and feed themselves. Incontinence was also a problem. Anyone who visits a poorly run nursing home will find many of these same conditions. There appears to be a "giving up" of the will to live by those who are deprived of caring touch.

Increased understanding of the importance of touch has changed even the way birth is handled. In the past, some mothers never touched their babies or even saw the newborn until he or she was cleaned up and made ready for display. Today parent-child "bonding" is considered an important part of the birth process and presents us with quite a different scene, a scene in which touching is given special attention.[6] Instead of being in the waiting room, the father is likely to witness the birthing and may even give a bit of assistance. Unless there is some complication, both parents can be in intimate physical contact with the baby immediately after it is born. It is believed that this close involvement creates a crucial bond between parent and child that will add to the quality of life for everyone.

"Truly, to touch is to give life."

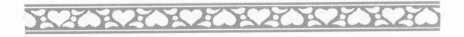

Sensitivity to Touch

The skin is the largest of the body's organs and serves a number of purposes. It enables us to sense the gentlest of breezes and wears rather well, considering the abuse it takes over a lifetime. We could be deaf, blind, and unable to smell or taste and still survive, but we could not live without the functions our skin carries out. Besides serving as a sense organ, the skin protects the inner body and is its temperature regulator. Of the sensory systems, the skin is the only one we cannot live without.

Although touch is known as the "mother of senses" because it is the first to develop, we mostly take it for granted. We expect to live for a lifetime distinguishing between sensations such as hot and cold, pain and pleasure. Accidents, illness, and age may diminish our touch sensitivity, but only in unusual cases does this sense disappear. Each of us has about eighteen square feet of skin filled with receptors waiting to accept messages to be transmitted to the brain through the nerves. Thanks to touch, vital information is available not only from the tips of our fingers (each of which has over 1,000 nerve endings) but from everywhere else on the body as well. On the average, a patch of skin the size of a quarter has twelve feet of nerves and twenty-five nerve endings, helping to make each one of us a self-contained communication network.

The skin is an early warning system that is quite sensitive even when we sleep. It recovers faster than other senses do when we awake.

Besides providing us with information, our sense of touch makes it possible to communicate without words. While we're still babies, most of us learn some of the different meanings communicated by touch. We discover that a kiss on the forehead is hardly the same as a slap on the backside and that a pinch of the arm says something quite different from a stroke of the shoulder. Our sense of touch can warn us of danger or tell us whether we're being punished or rewarded.

One of the first people to write extensively about the sense of touch was Ashley Montagu, who says:

> The differences between individuals in skin sensitivity are quite remarkable. There are some who when they touch another feel "a sort of electrical current" passing between them, whereas others experience nothing of the sort. It is also of interest to note that while some individuals retain this sensitivity into old age, others tend to lose it in middle age.[7]

In babies the sense of touch is the one most completely developed at birth. Other senses are much slower to develop. While many of the sense organs take up only a small portion of the body, the sense of touch is spread across the whole skin.

It's not known precisely what can be done to increase touch sensitivity, but it is clear that the level of sensitivity can be changed. The story of Helen Keller's life reveals how much of the world can be experienced through keen touch awareness. Massage therapists report an increased ability to feel and identify very small shapes with their fingertips and a heightened ability to distinguish slight changes in texture and temperature of the body. It may well be that what happens is simply a higher development of the touch potential we all have.

"Although touch is known as the 'mother of senses' because it is the first to develop, we mostly take it for granted."

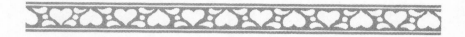

Fear of Touch

Despite the critical importance of touch most adult Americans remain reluctant to touch or be touched. Unfortunately, the sources of our reluctance are often well-meaning authority figures whose influence has had an ongoing impact on our lives that is difficult to overcome. When we were infants, our parents told us over and over, "Don't touch this!" "Don't touch that!" As we were growing up, we heard members of the clergy rail against the sins of the flesh, equating touch with sex and sin. Haven't we all watched doctors wash their hands immediately after touching us? The idea that we're "germy," "dirty," and "untouchable" is played up by advertisers who suggest we're all in need of deodorant from scalp to toe. In addition, we worry that someone may touch us and discover an imagined shortcoming in our anatomy. Zoologist Desmond Morris maintains that "Western society as a whole has retained its general mood of body-privacy and contact-taboo."[8]

In elevators we not only avoid touch but also conversation. In auditoriums, waiting rooms, churches, and other places where we normally sit, we tend to leave an empty seat between ourselves and the next person. We each want to have our own space, but having it can be a questionable luxury at times. During the height of the energy crisis in the seventies, Americans were so reluctant to give up the one-to-a-car mentality that many were willing to "fight it out" in gas lines in order to remain independent and untouchable.

On the other hand, there are circumstances under which we have such a zest to touch one another that we succumb to a kind of mob frenzy. The pileups of bodies squeezing, thumping, and hand slapping in games such as football and hockey are viewed by millions who consider this normal and natural activity. Men, who would not ordinarily put their arms around one another in other circumstances, appear to use sports to satisfy a need for touch.

Other events such as funerals momentarily set aside the touch taboo, allowing both men and women to hug, touch, pat, and stroke one another.

In sports, it is joy that gives free expression to touch. In funerals, it is sorrow. This suggests that during times of intense emotion it is natural, normal, and necessary to be in direct physical contact with another person.

The taboo against members of the same sex putting their arms around one another or walking hand in hand can be traced to fear of being labeled gay or lesbian. This is a persistent idea that causes much pain and prevents many of us from expressing our feelings through touch. Thirty years after it happened, a publishing executive still remembers when touching between himself and his father ended. During the confusing onset of puberty for the boy, his father— who up until then had always been a hugging, touching, tussling man—suddenly announced that they couldn't touch any more. Fortunately, this story of sense deprivation has a happy ending. That boy is now a man who makes sure his children are not deprived of the parental warmth and support that he had felt a great need for and been denied.

Indeed, we need to be set free of our reluctance to touch. In order to benefit fully from massage, examine your feelings about touching and being touched. Anxious feelings are real and to be respected. Try to resolve whatever reservations you may have and share your first massage experiences only with someone you trust.

"Indeed, we need to be set free of our reluctance to touch."

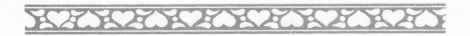

Touch Misused

Touching is a form of attention, and attention is something most people enjoy whether they are young or old. We know, however, that not all forms of touch are healthful and life-sustaining. Slapping, spanking, pinching, and punching are four common forms of hurtful touch that are too often administered by parents and teachers, some of whom quote Scripture in defense of their actions. When we listen carefully to the life stories of sensitive, thinking adults who grew up under the "spare the rod, spoil the child" rule, we hear sad, sad stories. It appears that negative touch seldom—if ever—leads to positive results.

Physically battered and sexually abused people of any age understand how touch can become a deadly weapon. Although some women do abuse touch, men do so more often. Commonly it is a relative—father, stepfather, grandfather, uncle, cousin, or even brother— who distorts the nourishing meaning of touch. An estimated six million wives are abused by their husbands in the United States each year.[9]

At any age, it is a devastating and dehumanizing experience to have a person you are supposed to trust and look to for guidance touch you in an unwanted way. For children, besides being overpowered and overwhelmed, there is the problem of feeling responsible, that it is their fault. Subsequently, some victims are unable to lead normal lives even after they become adults.

According to the American Humane Association, victimization of boys in the United States tripled from 1977 to 1981. One man who now works with such victims was himself abused (from age eleven through sixteen) by a family friend who was an adult leader of a youth group. The boy was made to feel that it was his fault because he was "demon-possessed."[10]

How insidious such an abuse of touch can be was explained by a marriage counselor who told of a case involving two sisters in their late forties. Each remained silent, thinking she was the only one abused by their father during childhood. If one of these women hadn't eventually sought help for a marital problem and been encouraged to speak up about everything troubling her, they both might have carried the secret to the grave. As it was, they broke their silence and discovered that their father had not only abused them but was now abusing their daughters. In this case, revealing their long-kept secret guilt enabled the sisters to take comfort from one another, put a stop to further abuse of the grandchildren, and act to minimize the damage.

Of course, touching can be done at the wrong time to the wrong person and in the wrong amount, but this should not prevent us from using the gift at those times when touch is an appropriate action. Touch should be soothing and assuring, a source of comfort and a means of building trust. If it is anything other than that, it is probably misused touch.

"Touch should be soothing and assuring, a source of comfort and a means of building trust."

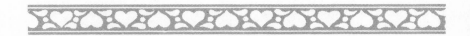

Sex and Massage

In the United States, the words "massage" and "parlor" are as commonly associated with one another as bread and butter, and legitimate massage therapists continue to struggle against guilt by association. The image of massage as an act involving sex and sin is one that catches the public's attention and leads to condemnation of the guilty and innocent alike. In St. Paul, Minnesota, even a Roman Catholic nun, Sister Rosalind Gefre, had a tussle with the law. In her youth, Rosalind Gefre personally experienced the cure of a painful ear condition through healing touch. This led eventually to her adult interest in touch and massage. Sister Rosalind and her associates challenged the city's massage parlor laws by refusing to apply for the then current city licenses when they opened their massage center in 1983.

Sister Rosalind and her associates believed that the laws were created to limit prostitution and did not apply to their Professional Massage Center. They were therapists, not call girls, and had no intention of giving up or giving in. Eventually, the licensing problem was resolved and the center stayed in business.[11] But the bigger problem remains in cities large and small. Honest, hard-working practitioners of the art of massage live under a cloud of dubious public opinion. The same thing was true in London in 1894. At that time, four women joined forces to try to make the massage profession "a safe, clean and honourable one for British women."[12] They ended up forming the Chartered Society of Physiotherapy but were unable to resolve the issue.

Today, with their reputations tainted, many masters of massage avoid advertising and don't set up their own public businesses. Instead, they either work quietly through established health spas and athletic clubs or go underground and accept clients strictly on a referral basis.

It's true that many massage and sauna parlors are fronts for various types of sexual activity, but these businesses would not exist if there weren't a demand. Investigation indicates, however, that it isn't simply sexual satisfaction clients are seeking. Is it surprising that many men are more *touch starved* than sex hungry? It isn't surprising to those who know that men and women are not so different when it comes to hunger for touch. Many women with a great desire to be held, cuddled, and caressed turn to prostitution because of unmet needs that can usually be traced back to childhood. Ashley Montagu makes this observation:

. . . in the Western world it is highly probable that sexual activity, indeed the frenetic preoccupation with sex that characterizes Western culture, is in many cases not the expression of a sexual interest at all, but rather a search for the satisfaction of the need for contact.[13]

Interviews with men reveal that many of them feel they have lived a lifetime of touch isolation, touching only while shaking hands or making love and have actually *never* experienced an extended period of giving or receiving non-sexual touch. For such men, the thought of gifting someone with even a five-minute massage is a threat to the way they have been brought up.

There also appears to be a widespread inability to make a distinction between sensuous touch and sexual touch. The result is more confusion about the legitimate uses of massage. Sensuous touch is what we feel through non-threatening massage when we are allowed to enjoy our body. This is the same feeling produced by warmth and water when you linger in a bath or by the warm sun and the breeze when you lie on the beach. Of course, it's true that the sensuous touch of massage *may* lead to an interest in sexual activity, *but it does not have to.* On the other hand, the goal of sexual touch is always some form of sexual activity.

Some people believe that women's liberation has had a direct influence on the growth in the number of massage parlors. The idea is suggested that men are afraid of assertive and independent women. There are others who feel that men and women—single or married—just don't communicate their needs to one another. There are also theories that imply that lax moral standards keep massage parlors in business or that it may be men's need for adventure or lack of self-esteem. While there may be some truth in all of these, Montagu's idea that meaningful touch is in all too short supply for everyone might well be the main reason. If so, the resolution of the massage parlor problem could be much closer to home than we realize.

"Sensuous touch is what we feel through non-threatening massage when we are allowed to enjoy our body."

Can the Hands Heal?

The "laying on" of hands to heal both the spiritual and the physical self is one of the oldest of rituals. Cave paintings made as long as 15,000 years ago depict the healing use of hands. Belief in the divine power of French and English kings to heal is well documented. The "king's hand" or "royal touch," an ability supposedly given to rulers by God, was an idea that enjoyed immense popularity among the people of that time. The English kept especially good records on the subject, reporting that in one year Edward I touched over 1,000 of his subjects who suffered from scrofula, a form of tuberculosis.[14] How many were actually healed is difficult to say, since there were few follow-up studies done in those days. The Reformation appears to have diminished the belief, perhaps because the idea of kings and saints performing miracle cures was repugnant to Protestants.

In our own time, faith healers have developed large followings. Many evangelists using TV as an electronic church suggest that miracle healings are commonplace and may even be experienced while kneeling in front of and touching the TV screen on which the healer appears. The fact is that such healings are difficult to document through any means other than word of mouth, which often tends to be exaggerated. There is no doubt, however, that many people are healed simply because they believe they are. This effect is similar to results obtained from the use of placebos. (People are healed by taking such things as sugar pills that they *believe* to be real medicine.) On the other hand, some members of the medical profession have done considerable investigation that tends to indicate that much laying on of hands and faith healing is a cruel hoax. William Nolen has investigated such cures as those brought about by the supposedly bloodless surgery performed in the Philippines.[15] In this case, the sleight of hand used to show supposed tissue removal is like that employed by the magician who pulls rabbits out of hats.

Still, touch does lead to healing. It isn't clear precisely how and why, but the age-long belief in healing hands is beginning to be scientifically documented. Of particular interest is the work of Dolores Krieger, who is a registered nurse and a professor. The nursing profession is unique in that touching is not only a legitimate function of the profession but also an integral part of the plan to help and heal. Although Krieger has done lengthy studies that are difficult to summarize, her concept of Therapeutic Touch has roots in the ancient laying on of hands. Her contact with the healer Oskar Estebany led her into an extended study of touching with the intent to heal. Krieger learned the process of healing by the laying on of hands from Dora Van Gelder Kunz. Krieger says, "The healees would feel heat in the tissues underlying the area over which I held my hands; they would feel profoundly relaxed; and they reported a sense of well-being."

Krieger's work is being replicated and extended. Therapeutic Touch is now being taught at the university level. Those who use it with the intent to help and heal report very specific results. There is an immediate drop of several decibels in the voice, and breathing becomes slower and deeper. There is an audible sigh of relaxation and a slight pinking of the skin. One of the interesting things Krieger has discovered is that the person in need of healing need not exhibit a religious belief in order to experience the effect of a healing touch that has the intent to help.[16]

"The age-long belief in healing hands is beginning to be scientifically documented."

Giving the Gift
of Massage

In New York a massage can cost fifty dollars or more, and clients such as dancers, who depend on massage to overcome muscle cramping and various types of minor injuries, are often reluctant to reveal the names of their masseuses or masseurs for fear that they will soon be overbooked. At least one dance company has a Swedish masseur on its payroll to keep its performers in condition. It's reported that five minutes of massage can restore tired muscles up to 100 percent, whereas five minutes of rest restores them only about twenty percent.[17] The rejuvenation that dancers experience through therapeutic massage is welcomed by other people as well, including Neil Simon, Bette Midler, and Jackie Onassis.

What others pay to receive, you can give for free. The loving touch of your hands is a gift of immeasurable worth that can benefit your friend, spouse, child, parent, or lover.

As you begin to give massages, you'll become aware of a feeling of energy within yourself. It's a synergistic experience in which the total effect appears greater than the individual effects. One man who was just learning massage explained, "At first I was a little nervous about the whole thing. I was afraid maybe I wouldn't do it right. When I started, it just seemed natural and I realized how connected I felt. I didn't expect it, but something really good was happening to me too."

Touching is such a personal experience that it can bring forth quite unexpected results. For example, massaging a child may bring back memories of your own childhood or, if you are a parent, memories of your child's birth and younger years. You might feel tearful and joyful at one and the same time as you recall personal and meaningful moments.

One of the few things we can give the elderly that is of real value to them is our presence made real through touch. If you sit quietly at the bedside of someone you love who is confined to a nursing home and gently massage that person's hand, you may be overwhelmed by emotion. You may become angry at yourself for having waited so long to share your tender touch. Or your usual reluctance to talk freely may be overcome, and you might find yourself open to discussion of something that had previously been hidden like a skeleton in a closet. It's almost as though physical contact frees people to be more open in expressing and exploring what it means to have life and be "in touch" with another person.

Touch is not an emotion, but it creates the changes within our bodies that we label emotions. Men who learn how to give massages often report sensing great feelings of tenderness when they break through the no-touch barriers they've lived with for a lifetime. Those who have grown up thinking of themselves as "takers" may be surprised by their ability to give without expecting something in return.

Our first language is touch, and if we don't learn it well in our early years we may never become expert at it. We can, however, develop the ability to be less "touchy" about what we don't know and learn how to both give and receive more supportive and loving touches.

I have separated the Swedish massage for the entire body into a series of easy-to-give massages that you can master one by one. As your skill and confidence increase, you can combine more and more of the massages until you're able to do the complete sequence.

"The loving touch of your hands is a gift of immeasurable worth that can benefit your friend, spouse, child, parent, or lover."

Massage and Exercise

In the past decade, millions of us have taken up some physical activity on a regular basis. Runners jog their way along even the busiest city streets and health clubs have become social centers as well as places to work out. Concern for health has become a lifestyle, and all the beautiful people have written exercise books that include sections on everything from makeup to diet. Fitness is much more than a passing fad, but just how is it best attained and then maintained? And what role can massage play? Although a few experts had questioned the long range value of strenuous workouts, it was only after running expert Jim Fixx died while jogging that the real worth of exercise began to be examined. Researchers couldn't seem to trot out their opinions fast enough, and studies were quickly released to illuminate one point or another. The conclusions regarding what is and isn't good for us will long be argued.

In the meantime, we know that our bodies were made to move. There's no question about it. Long ago people exercised all day as part of their physical labors. Today a great many of us live such sedentary lives behind desks and at computer terminals that we have to swim, dance, lift weights, play tennis, or do some other physical activity on a regular schedule in order to balance inaction with action and maintain such important qualities as body flexibility, muscle tone, and even correct posture. But along with getting the blood flowing and the lungs heaving, exercise changes the chemistry of the body and often leaves us with stiff muscles, cramps, and even constipation. Besides that, bruised parts of our system need healing. This is where the art of Swedish massage has a definite role to play in overall well-being. I believe that anyone who is participating in a physical fitness program—in either a casual or a purposeful way—should include the use of massage. It's a health-maintaining tool. Why not use it?

It's not necessary to know much about anatomy when you're first learning how to give a Swedish massage. You should, however, have at least some sense of what goes on inside the body when it's stroked and tapped and vibrated after exercise.

The massage movements that feel so good against the skin are actually changing our inner workings. Nerves are stimulated both near the surface of the skin and deep within the body, blood flow is enhanced, and so is the movement of lymph. Among many other things, the increased blood flow supplies oxygen where it's needed and gets nutrients into the lymph fluid and on its way to individual cells. Swedish massage therapists often speak about the "lymph draining" that accompanies a full body massage. The lymph doesn't drain away in the sense that sweat and urine do. Rather, its rate of flow is increased.

Lymph is a colorless fluid that flows through vessels in a system similar to the blood circulatory system. The makeup of lymph includes water, white blood cells, digested food, waste given off by the body, and various other substances. Lymph is extremely important because it nourishes and bathes the body cells and helps to rid the body of wastes produced during exercise. Most of us are familiar with lymph nodes. They are, in effect, tiny filters that break down waste products into chemicals the blood can carry away to the kidneys for elimination. The nodes are the connections between the lymph system and the blood system. If there were only the blood system, an infection could be carried to the entire body in minutes. The major lymph nodes are located in the abdomen and chest, so massaging these areas has a direct impact on the whole lymphatic system. I don't recommend that you massage any one area of the body on an exclusive basis. The Swedish massage techniques are meant to be used from foot to head, so that the entire body can benefit.

Of course there are times when a particular part of the body is literally calling for help. I remember especially a day when I had my portable massage table set up near the finish line of a marathon. The race had been run on a cloudless day with a constantly rising temperature, and many of the runners were suffering from dehydration despite their intake of water along the route of the marathon. One runner had such severe leg cramps that he was moaning in great pain and had to be assisted onto my table. This was not the time or place for a full body massage. I worked immediately on his legs and soon rid him of excruciating cramps. In such a case, the person giving the massage can actually feel the knotting muscles release and relax. The reason I remember that day so well is because the newspaper printed a picture of me at work. The picture was taken near the runner's contorted face and gave newspaper readers the impression that I was inflicting the pain rather than easing it!

After a major run, many runners wait for up to two weeks for their bodies to recuperate before beginning training for a next run. With massage, this recuperation time can often be shortened to a few days.

If health and an all-over feeling of wellness are important to you, you've probably already made a lot of choices regarding diet, vitamins, and exercise. You probably feel that you're in control of your destiny and are pleased with yourself. After all, you're doing what you believe is good for you. That's great, but unless you're very unusual you've probably missed a major beneficial activity. Massage. You can do some of it on yourself, but for the full benefit, you have to find someone else who will do it for you. Believe me, if you put yourself in someone else's hands, lie back and accept a full body Swedish massage, you'll wonder why you waited so long to discover the magic of this ancient art.

Why not get a partner and learn together?

"The massage movements that feel so good against the skin are actually changing our inner workings."

PART · TWO

Preparing
for
Massage

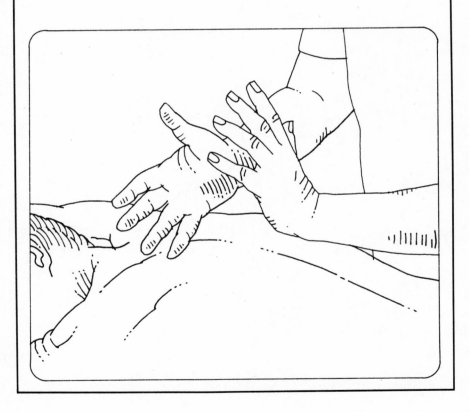

Oils and Creams

Any type of vegetable oil or fine mineral oil that will remain thin—and not get sticky—may be used to enhance the touches and strokes of Swedish massage. Of the vegetable oils, olive oil, almond oil, safflower oil, and coconut oil are particularly recommended because they are easily available and stay fluid enough to allow the proper friction for massage. There is considerable evidence and knowledgeable opinion that natural oils provide nourishment for the skin. For scenting, concentrated oils such as lemon oils, rose oils, and many of the flavoring oils found on the cooking spice shelves in grocery stores can be mixed with the more bland vegetable oils to enhance the aromatic effects of massage. Vegetable oils have some disadvantages. They are relatively expensive, and some tend to thicken after being heated, requiring unused oil to be thrown out. You may also find that many people have skin that is sensitive to some oils.

Certain types of mineral oil are made especially for use on the skin. Although baby oil can be used for massage, it is rather thick, and extra oil has to be added frequently to keep it liquid enough. This disturbs the rhythm that makes a good massage. Use of any thick oil is a distinct disadvantage in the massage of very hairy persons where extra oil must be used to avoid pulling the hair out by the friction of the hands on the skin. Some massage therapists advance the opinion that mineral oils clog the pores and harm the skin. This opinion appears to be without any verifiable basis in fact. What is true, however, is that many purists sell their own "mix" of oils at prices ranging up to fifty dollars per gallon, whereas mineral oils range from eight to twenty dollars per gallon.

Mineral oils have been used by countless mothers on their babies without adverse effects. A simple toweling with a damp terrycloth towel or a warm shower following the massage will remove the oil.

I have used a special thin form of mineral oil, called white oil, for more than ten years with never an instance of skin irritation or customer complaint. Many bakeries use this oil to grease baking pans, because it is pure and inexpensive. To prevent contamination, this oil can be shipped only in new barrels. It is so thin it will actually evaporate, leaving no residue on the bakery products and little, if any, residue on the skin. If you're a good bakery customer, your baker may be induced to sell you some of this oil. Up to twelve dollars is a fair price for a gallon. The alternative is to buy directly from a petroleum products warehouse. Amoco makes this type of oil under various names and/or number codes. One of the names is White Rose Oil.

This white oil is hypo-allergenic, gets thinner as it gets warmer, and, by using more or less, you can maintain a precise measure of hand friction. The oil can be scented by adding any perfume, cologne, or flavoring you desire, although some scents do not mix as well and require frequent shaking or stirring. *A much more effective method is to gently rub a scented body oil onto the body before or after applying the unscented massage oil.*

I save empty dishwashing detergent bottles with pull-up stoppers for later use as oil dispensers. When well-rinsed, they make excellent oil bottles, but the contents should be marked on the bottles to prevent accidental use for some other purpose. Bottled oil is easily heated in a large pan of hot water (never on a stove or in an oven or microwave) or by placing a *full* bottle, with its stopper open, on a ceramic dish about six inches in front of an electric room heater. (The bottle should be full to prevent the plastic from melting.) Don't use a baby bottle warmer because it could be as dangerous to use as a stove. A plastic bottle can melt and the oil can burn. *Never use glass containers.* Glass of any kind should be kept out of the massage area, shower, and bathroom. Broken glass can cut feet and tiny shards may be all but impossible to remove from some types of carpeting.

If no other method is available for heating oil, it may be heated to a comfortable temperature by merely holding it cupped in your palm. Whether the oil is warm or cold, I often pour it directly from the squirt bottle through the back of the knuckles of one of my hands and onto the person I'm massaging. The knuckles act as tiny radiators, cooling or warming the oil to body temperature, as needed.

The oils I've mentioned may be used for the entire body but there are certain special oils that, if available, should be used on the face, the hands and feet, and those areas of the body with especially delicate skin, particularly areas where the wearing of synthetic fiber fabrics has impaired the ability of the skin to "breathe" (eliminate waste through perspiration). The skin is one of the major organs for the elimination of body waste, along with the lungs and kidneys, and is also the body's main temperature controller. Synthetic fiber clothing, the sun, and the wind play a large part in aging the skin. Special oils containing ingredients such as cocoa butter, lanolin, aloe vera, and vitamins A, D, and E will often improve damaged skin. Careful massage can also play a role in reducing the visible effect of skin damage. Some of the Swedish techniques are so effective that the results on any part of the body, in terms of color and tone, are often immediate and clearly visible.

There are many facial creams available that contain some or all of the above ingredients that may be of benefit when used on the more delicate skin areas. Some soak in so quickly that additional cream is required during the massage. I prefer to work in a room that's warm enough to bring a sheen of perspiration to the skin. This helps keep any good cream moist and allows me to continue working instead of stopping to apply more cream. Don't ever buy oil or cream on the basis of cost alone. Testing a variety of products will help you decide which suits you best. I have found that the following are readily available and of high quality:

- Vitamin E Moisture Lotion by Nature's Finest, made by Walgreen Labs of Chicago and sold by Walgreens Drugstores, often at a "two-for-one-cent-more sale."
- Shaklee's Skin Conditioner called Tioga, made from Shaklee's special oils and herbs and available through Shaklee distributors.
- Golden Harvest Hand and Body Lotion, available at all General Nutrition Corporation stores.

These three are the best I have found for the face, chest, shoulder, and upper leg areas that are most often exposed to the elements or synthetic fiber clothing.

For the hands and feet, there are many creams and lotions available that contain the above ingredients, but nothing I have found comes close to Shaklee's minty Medicated Foot Creme. It softens corns and calluses and kills germs. This cream might more aptly be labeled "hand and foot" cream because it soothes the skin of the foot you're working on as well as the skin of your own hands, leaving the skin strong, pliable, and soft as suede glove leather.

It is absolutely essential that both the massagee's and the massager's nails be close-clipped and smooth. The "Trim" brand offers a most efficient fingernail clipper and also a special toenail clipper with a convex cutting edge that will help prevent ingrown toenails.

Precautions

Precautions, which massage therapists refer to as "contra-indications to massage," include medical reasons for limiting massage as well as common sense rules regarding hygiene and general care of the body. My list of precautions for the massages described is not all-inclusive, but those I mention apply to the general art of massage. They are guidelines anyone interested in massage should be aware of. Many instruction books ignore this area altogether. I believe it is important for everyone to understand that there are instances when massage should be avoided and other times when it should be done only with special knowledge and extra care.

Hygiene

Before beginning a massage, you should be aware of any medical history that may be pertinent. (See specifics later in this section.)

If you're going to combine a number of the massage techniques from this book, a sauna or warm bath or shower before the massage is beneficial. (See section on Hot and Cold Techniques.)

Many people suffer from athlete's foot. Germicidal sprays and powders are available for use on rugs and shower and sauna floors. I recommend Desenex powder for the feet.

All cloth materials used during massage can be easily disinfected by adding a half a cup of ordinary bleach to the laundry wash water.

Guidelines

You should not do any massage if you have any active illness or an unhealed injury on your hands.

- Massage is not recommended for anyone who is obviously sick—feverish, continuously sneezing or coughing, etc. (Professionals require a doctor's written approval in hand.)

- Avoid foot massage on anyone suffering from athlete's foot.

- Avoid massaging any area sore or swollen with arthritis-like pain.

- Do not massage anyone who has skin cancer, leukemia, or Hodgkin's Disease. (For massage of anyone having other types of cancer, professionals require a doctor's written approval in hand.)

- Do not do frontal body massage on anyone who has had abdominal surgery within the past six months.

- Do not massage a diabetic's legs or the legs of anyone suffering from inflamed varicose veins, phlebitis, or other blood vessel problems. Warning signs are ulcers, swollen or inflamed veins, or numerous black and blue marks on the arms or legs. (These may indicate weakened blood vessels.)

- Avoid massaging the abdomen of anyone suffering from high blood pressure, unless medical treatment has corrected it to normal range.
- Massage should always be stopped six inches on either side of a recent wound, sore, or inflamed area.
- Any forceful massage stroke should always be done toward the heart.
- Women should avoid abdominal or forceful lower back massage during the first two days of their period or during pregnancy.
- Do not massage anyone with general edema (the whole body is noticeably swollen with excessive body fluid). Pressing the skin of a person with this condition will often leave a dent, so the condition is easily recognized.
- Some people have swelling of the knees, ankles, belly, or buttocks caused by fluid retention and may be massaged but only with a very gentle, flowing stroke.

Massage Accessories

Practically all massage can be done with nothing more than a pair of gentle hands, a bottle of oil, and a terrycloth towel. A few additional items are useful and can be acquired as time goes on: a stereo or a good radio tuned to a music station, preferably playing very soft mood music; an electric heater to warm the room and the oil; an electric vibrating massage machine. (I've found the two-handed type made by Morfam, Inc., of Mishawaka, Indiana, to be highly dependable, but any similar type will do.) If you're going to do massage on a regular basis, you'll find a couple of bolsters twenty-four inches long, eight to twelve inches in diameter, very helpful. They go under the knees of the person being massaged when lying face up or under the ankles when the person is lying face down. Use of a bolster will reduce the muscle tension in the thighs and lower back. (A pillow will serve the same purpose.) One or more U-shaped, neck support pillows will make breathing more comfortable for a person lying face down. These are arranged in various positions under the forehead and chin.

You can make a massage platform by lining up couch cushions on the floor and covering them first with a thick, folded blanket and then adding a soft sheet. A table, of course, is much better. A five- to six-foot-long banquet table with folding legs makes a very effective surface, particularly if you cover it with a fairly dense two-inch foam pad. Cover that with a sheet of vinyl and a cloth sheet. (An exercise mat will also serve well.) The table can be stored on end behind a door or in a closet when not in use. The pad can be stored beneath a bed or sofa. When using a table with folding legs, be sure they are sturdy enough to support a person and have locking pins on the legs to prevent accidents. (I always reinforce the locks on my portable tables with a strong duct tape each time I set them up.)

If you have the room for a permanent table and want to build a sturdy one, you can find excellent table plans in *The Massage Book* by George Downing.

Hot and Cold Techniques

Bathing
A warm, soaking bath or shower before a massage will open and cleanse the pores. Some of the fluids

released from the cells by the massage will flow outward through the skin rather than inward to the blood and kidneys. A full body, lymph and blood draining Swedish massage may send one to three pounds of waste fluid through the skin rather than the kidneys.

A sauna and a fairly hot shower before a massage and a hot shower slowly turned to a cold shower after the massage will enhance the effects of any massage and is especially recommended for those receiving a full body massage.

Sauna Tips
Some apparently healthy people are uncomfortable taking a sauna and may feel faint or dizzy. When that's the case, it's often helpful to wrap a cold wet towel around the neck and sip cool water or fruit juice during the sauna. Those who sauna regularly report that grapefruit juice increases sweating.

Certain water-soluble vitamins and minerals can be lost through excessive sweating. Anyone using a sauna more than once a week should be aware of this and take whatever vitamins and minerals may be necessary.

Cold and Hot Wetpacks
When you use alternate cold and hot wetpacks, the effect is similar to that when you flex your muscles. Bloodflow is stimulated.

To prepare wetpacks, you need two pails of water, one with cold and one with hot water. Add no more than a tray of ice cubes to the cold water. Soak one medium-size terrycloth towel in each pail. You have to work quickly in order to retain the heat and cold as you wring and place the towels. If your hands are strong enough, you may be able to fold the towels into packs before you soak them and wring them out. Otherwise, wring and fold the towel as quickly as you can. You *should apply the cold wetpack first* for thirty seconds or longer and follow with a hot wetpack for ten to twenty seconds. Continue alternating these applications for up to ten minutes.

Wetpacks are an effective, temporary remedy for most muscle aches and cramps, particularly when followed by a massage. Swelling from bumps and bruises can often be reduced to the point where a very gentle massage is permissible. No massage closer than six inches to an injured area should ever be given if the swelling is caused by a sprain, tendon damage, or an obvious infection.

Cold Water Soaks
Swelling of the feet, hands, arms, and legs may be relieved by soaking them in a pail or tub filled with cold water. You may want to add a little ice but don't make it into an ice bath. Gentle massage is permitted three to five days after minor injuries if there is no discoloration of the skin, but never directly on the injured area itself.

For a very sore back or other body area, an initially warm, shallow bath is beneficial. Immerse the sore area in the warm bath and then let the cold water run slowly until the bathwater has turned cold. Five minutes of cold soaking followed by a brief warm shower will often give relief.

As always, any condition that does not respond to the above should be referred to a medical doctor.

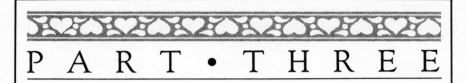

P A R T · T H R E E

Basic
Hand Positions
and Strokes

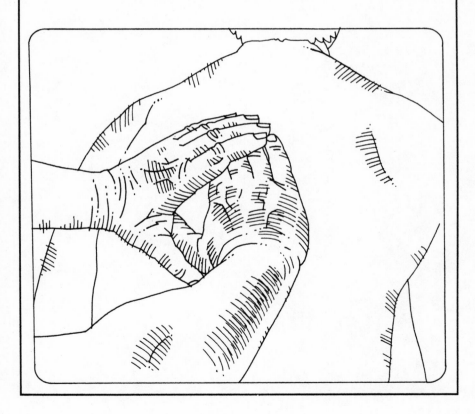

There should be no undue pain from massage. Always instruct the person you are massaging to inform you of any sore spots so that you may adjust the pressure of your stroke. Go lighter over sore spots and massage for a longer period.

It is possible to exert considerable pressure through flow strokes that involve the palm of the hand, but even greater, localized pressure can be exerted with the fingertips. The pressure of fingertip massage is transmitted through all the tissue, nerves, and blood vessels to the underlying bone. It's important to remember that we massage people to help them rather than hurt them. Although nerves tend to be buried deep in the tissue alongside bones, where they are protected, pressure improperly applied can injure them. Always ask for feedback from people you're massaging to help you apply pressure without causing pain.

For best results, the person you're massaging should do nothing to help except what you specifically ask for: "Turn over now," "Lift your arm," etc.

We are all physically different, so it's important as you learn to give massages that you be creative in your thinking. "Use what you have to do the best you can" is the rule to follow. This may require you to adapt some of the directions to fit your own strengths and weaknesses. You may find, for example, that you can use the backs of your bent knuckles in place of your fingertips for some of the petrissage strokes. If you have a weak arm or are missing a finger or have a dominant hand, experiment until you find a comfortable method of applying the required strokes, and you will be successful.

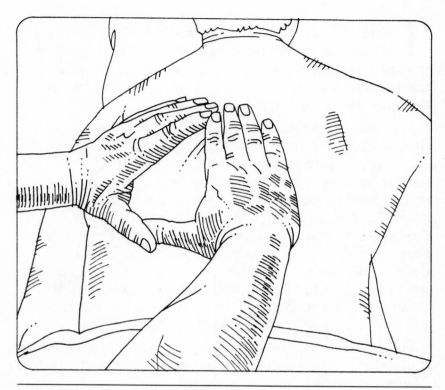

1. **Effleurage:** Large Christmas Tree

This stroke is used for spreading oil and generally warming the skin. It soothes and relaxes. Done gently, it can be used in any direction in much the same way you would move your hand when applying suntan lotion to someone's back.

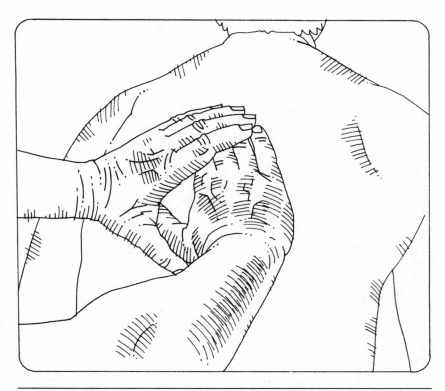

2. **Effleurage:** Small Christmas Tree

The hand position for the small Christmas tree allows for the application of considerable pressure. This is a power stroke and must always be done toward the heart. Remember to release the pressure at the end of the stroke and "trail back" your hands so that you retain skin contact.

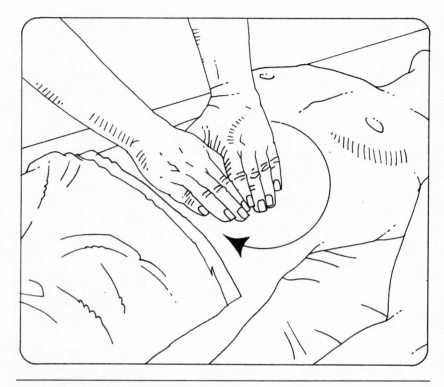

3. Effleurage: Clockwise

In Swedish massage, this stroke is used only on the
abdomen. It is done clockwise in order to follow the
direction of peristaltic action. Apply the stroke with even
pressure and move your hands slowly. Properly used, this
stroke can be done even on a person who is ticklish in the
abdominal area.

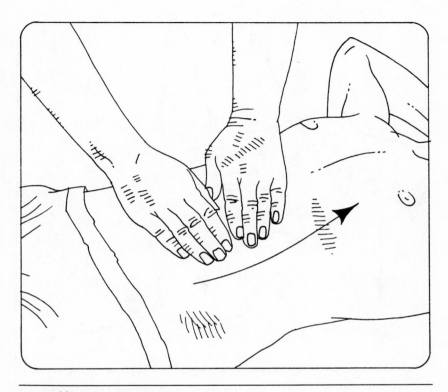

4. Effleurage: Sideways

This is a sweeping stroke in which your hands (or fingertips) release pressure at the end of the sweep and "trail back" so that you don't lose skin contact. This sideways stroke is used on the abdomen and chest.

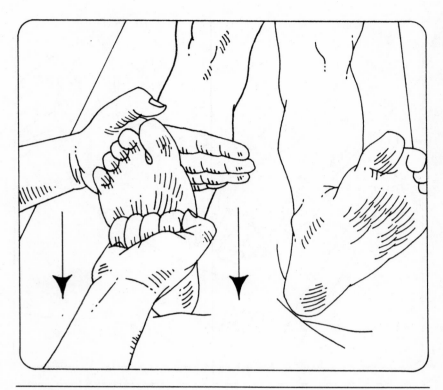

5. Effleurage: Knuckle

To form your hand properly for this stroke, extend your hand palm up and make a fist. The knuckle stroke is used on the sole of the foot. Always stroke the knuckles from toe to heel (toward the heart because this is a power stroke). As you stroke from toe to heel, the palm of your other hand must follow down the top of the foot for support.

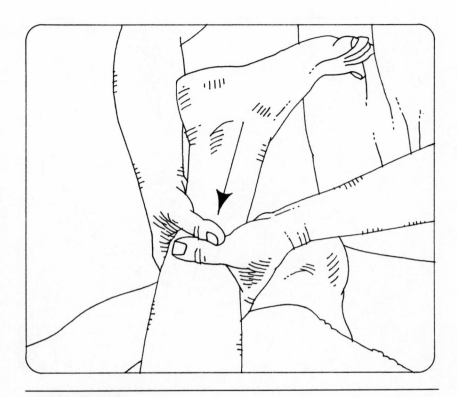

6. Wringing

This procedure is used to drain excess lymph, blood, and other fluids from the tissue. In wringing, you place your fingers and thumbs in "rings" around an arm or leg. Maintain even pressure as you slide the rings toward the torso. On the arms, slide from wrist to shoulder and on the legs, slide from ankle to the upper leg. (Wringing is always done toward the heart.) When you release your grip, trail your fingers back to the starting point. On a large arm or leg, encircle the limb as completely as you can with both hands and proceed as instructed above.

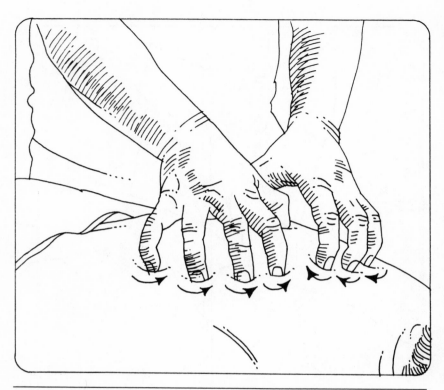

7. Petrissage: Two Hand and One Hand

This circular stroke is done with the fingers and thumbs spread and curled as though holding a softball. (Your fingernails should be closely trimmed.) The entire hand is rotated to move the fingertips and thumbtips on the skin in dime-size circles. (You may move your wrist a little, but mostly you move the whole arm at the elbow and shoulder. This enables you to maintain even pressure and cuts down on fatigue.) When using two hands, the left moves clockwise and the right counterclockwise. Two hands are used wherever the body surface is large enough. This circular stroke may be heavy or light and need not be toward the heart.

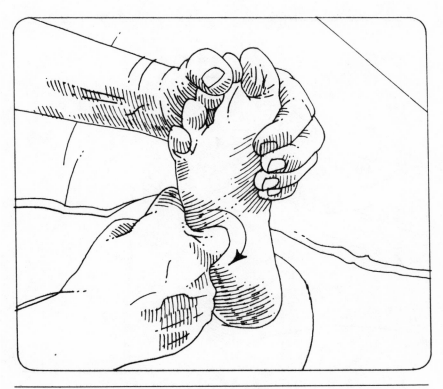

8. Petrissage: Knuckle "V"

This is used on small areas. It's most commonly used on
the edges of the foot where it enables you to keep good
contact control and not slip off. Always use your other
hand directly on the opposite side of the foot for support.
A person should not have to strain against the pressure you
apply. Although foot sensitivity varies, you should always
apply as much pressure as the person can comfortably stand.

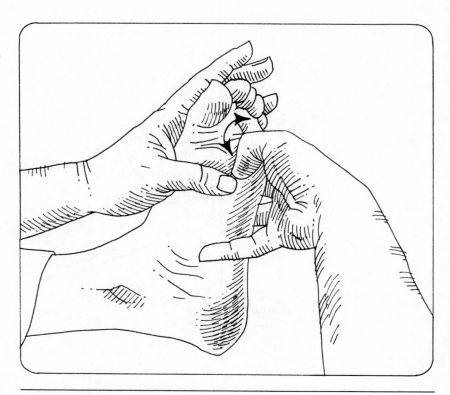

9. Petrissage: Thumb Tip or Thumb Knuckle

This stroke is used where you need a precise point for
application of pressure, especially on the bottom of the foot
and the palm of the hand. You may also find it useful on
the upper back and shoulder blade areas.

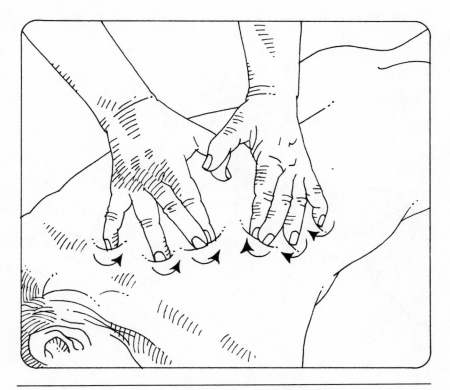

10. Petrissage: Overlapping Fingers

The overlapping of the fingers allows the same increased
pressure and control as when using the thumb. It is used
mainly on acupressure points on shoulders, upper back and
neck, and buttocks. (On heavily muscled or overweight
people, massage therapists sometimes even use the elbow.)
The illustration shows how to overlap both thumbs and
fingers. Use one method *or* the other.

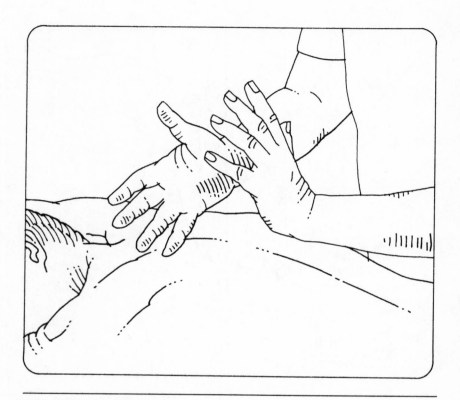

11. Hacking

This vibrating motion causes considerable nerve stimulation and reaches deep tissue. Hacking (and cupping) will bring a blush to the skin surface. Although it may look something like a series of quick judo chops, it's not! Hacking requires a drum-like tapping in which *only the tips of the little fingers contact the skin.* It is done with fingers held straight out and spread apart. (They will tap one against the other as your little fingers make contact with the skin.) During the hacking motions, you make alternate contact with your hands. It is done on the back of the calf, the upper leg, the buttocks, and back but *not* on the spine.

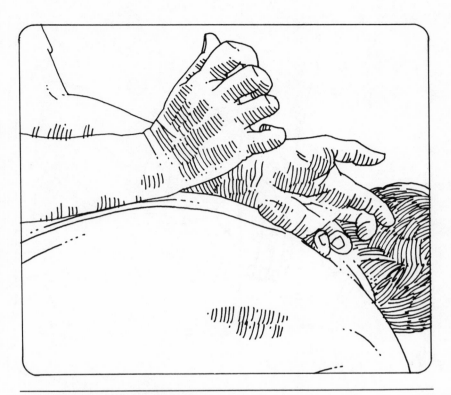

12. German Hammer

The German hammer involves striking with the loosely curved little finger *and* the fleshy edge of the palm. Note that it differs from hacking. The German hammer is used on the back of the body, mainly on the buttocks and the heavy muscle area of the upper shoulders. Never use on the kidney area.

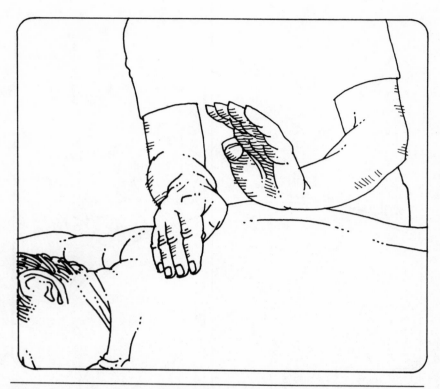

13. Cupping (with oil on bare skin only)

Successful cupping begins with the way you hold your
hands. The thumbtips are folded in under the base of the
index fingers and all the fingers are held slightly curled or
"cupped." Cupping is done on the back of the calf, the
upper leg, the buttocks, and back but *not* on the spine.
The curve of the cupped hands must follow the curve of
the body to prevent stinging with the fingertips. Strike
alternately with your hands and *draw them back immediately.*
This action momentarily sucks up the skin just as suction
cups would and causes greatly increased blood flow to the
skin.

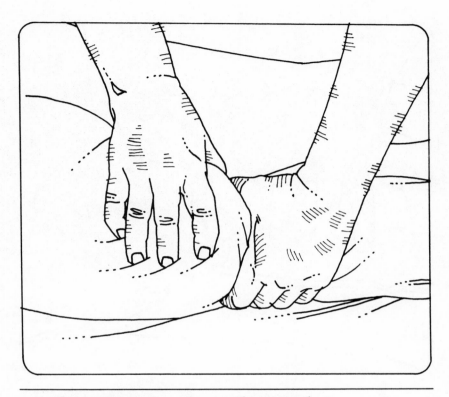

14. Kneading (on bare skin with or without oil)

Kneading involves friction. You knead only where there is ample tissue. Do not knead thin arms, legs, or other portions of the body where there is little tissue covering the underlying bone. To knead on bare skin, grasp tissue with both hands and roll it between them. This is done most successfully on the back of the calf, the entire upper leg, buttock, back, and arm.

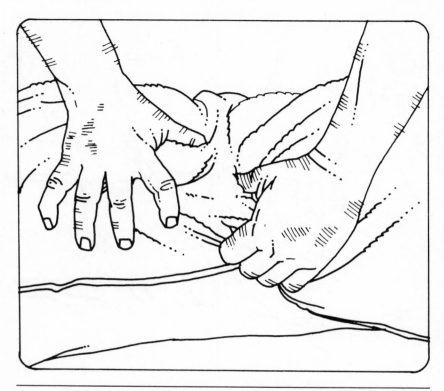

15. Kneading (through a towel)

This is especially effective on large fleshy areas. Cover the bare skin with a terrycloth towel. (If there is a coarse side to the towel, put that side down on the skin.) Grasp and release, move your hands slightly, grasp and release again. Do this rhythmically and continue until the area is covered. Be sure that you are grasping the flesh and not pinching it.

PART · FOUR

The Full Body
Swedish Massage

The following pages include easy-to-give massages that anyone, even a child, can give. They require no great strength. All you need is a warm and gentle touch and the desire to help. I have separated each massage into simple steps that you can learn quickly. As you become more experienced, you will be able to combine one massage with another and eventually give a full body Swedish massage that begins with the feet and works up the body to the top of the head.

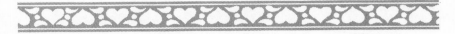

The Feet

The massage of the feet is done with oil, but first the feet should be washed. Warm water is most relaxing, but cool or even cold water is best for refreshing overworked feet. To soften calluses and remove dry skin, use a stiff, short-bristled brush and hot, soapy water.

Precautions
Don't massage anyone who has symptoms of athlete's foot (cracked, reddened, or peeling skin between the toes). Watch for symptoms of gout and arthritis (swollen and/or reddened skin). You should, in fact, ask whether the person suffers from either of these. Avoid massaging any afflicted area.

Although this is a simple massage, it is so pleasing that you should set aside plenty of time. Ticklishness can be lessened by beginning at the ankle and by avoiding too light a touch. Don't pull on the big toe. It can easily be pulled out of joint and is not easily put back! Rotate it gently instead.

Position
The person to be massaged lies face up on a firm bed or other massage surface. (If you're only doing the feet, the person can sit back in a comfortable chair while you sit to one side of the person's foot on a low chair or hassock.) Work on one foot at a time. The person's ankle should rest comfortably across your leg just above your knee.

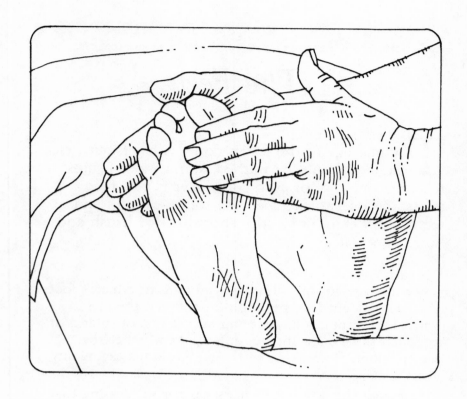

Sequence

1. Apply a high-quality, medicated foot cream. (See section on oils and creams.) Massage the cream into the skin with gentle effleurage.

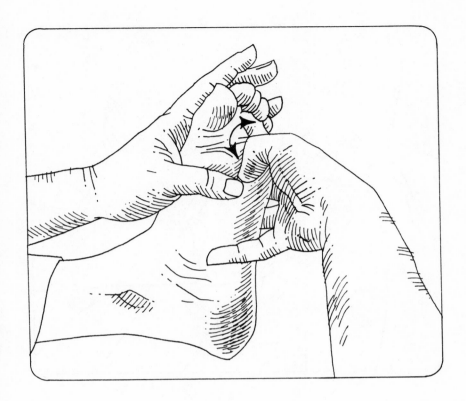

2. Use one hand to support the foot directly behind the spot you are massaging. To do the bottom of the foot, petrissage with one knuckle. Do 2-3 dime-size circles. Then, while retaining skin contact, slide your knuckle about one-half inch farther and repeat the petrissage, following this pattern:

Do the toes.

Do the ball of the foot.

Do the center of the foot.

Do the heel, including the sides up as far as the ankle bone.

You can repeat the toe-to-heel massage several times.

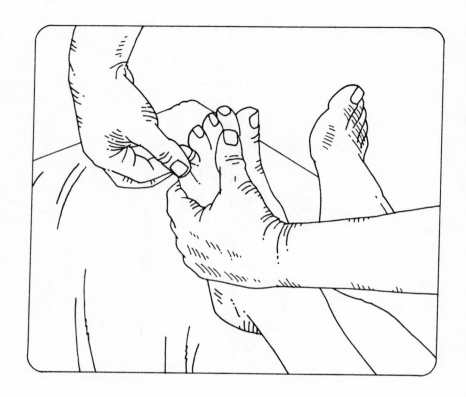

3. Pull and gently rotate each of the four toes (but *not* the big toe). There should be no pain. Don't be alarmed, however, if you hear a slight "click" or "snap." (What occurs is similar to what happens when you pull a finger to crack a knuckle.)

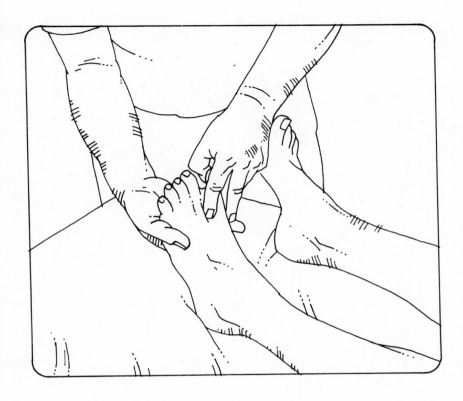

4. To do the top of the foot, use only the tip of the index finger to petrissage between the bones. *Be gentle.* The top of the foot includes many nerves and may be extremely sensitive. Begin at the base of the toes and work toward the ankle. Do the entire area once.

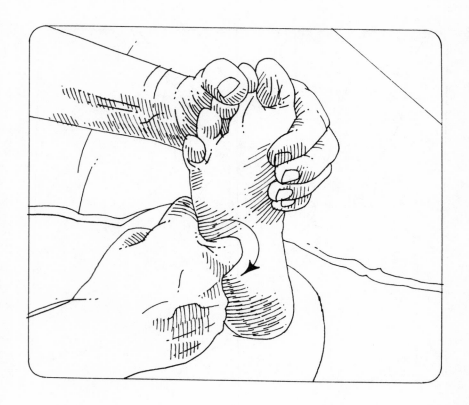

5. To do the inner and outer edges of the foot, support the foot with one hand and massage the upper and lower surfaces of the edge at the same time, with the knuckle V position. Begin making the dime-size circles at the base of the toe and work all the way to the heel and then up over the ankle. Do both edges.

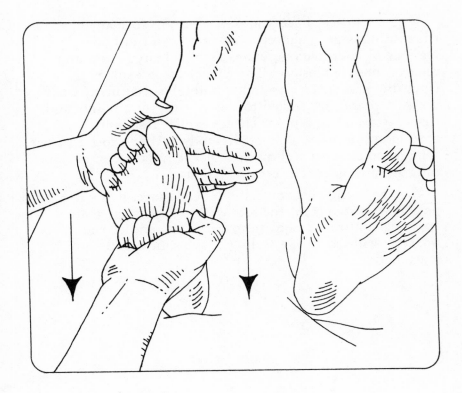

6. Make a fist with your massaging hand, palm upward. Support the opposite surface of the foot with your other hand as you effleurage with the middle knuckles of your closed hand. Make firm knuckle strokes on the bottom of the foot from the toes to the heel, 3-6 times, with the supporting hand following down the top of the foot so your hands remain opposite one another.

7. Repeat Steps #1-6 on the other foot.

When your feet hurt, you hurt all over. In many cases, the foot massage is almost as effective as a full body massage. A foot massage increases blood circulation and removes muscle tension. The theory of reflexology (pressure massage of foot reflex points) is that many body pressure points are related to the foot pressure points and that massage of one point creates similar results in corresponding parts all over the body. After a foot massage, some people report feeling that they're walking on air and can't seem to get their feet on the ground.

You can easily give yourself a foot massage. If you're a person who stands on the job, washing, massaging, and applying soothing oils to your feet at the end of the workday will result in a feeling of relaxation and rejuvenation.

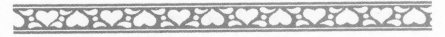

The Front of the Legs

Precautions
Do not massage the legs of anyone suffering from phlebitis, diabetes, or inflamed varicose veins. Signs to arouse caution include scars, unhealed sores, or large discolored veins. Always ask the person about any illness or injuries because many potential problems are not necessarily visible, especially when you can see only the front of the legs.

Position
The person to be massaged will lie face up on a firm bed or other massage surface. For comfort, place a small pillow under the head and a bolster beneath the knees.

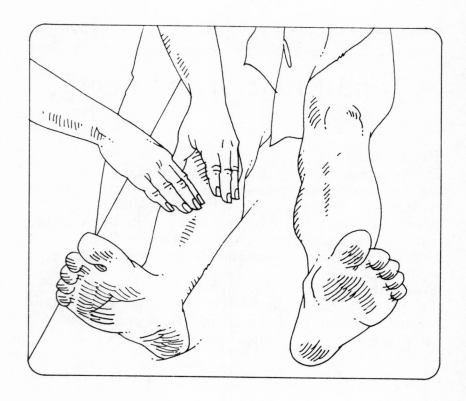

Sequence

1. Spread oil on top of *both* legs with a gentle stroke such as you would use to apply suntan lotion.

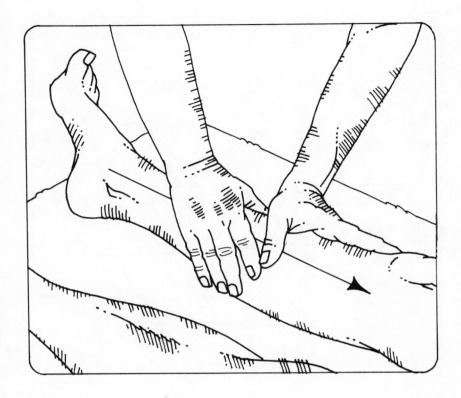

2. Begin with the right leg. (Do a complete massage of one leg before moving to do the other leg.) Effleurage from the ankle to the upper thigh. Maintain skin contact as you lightly draw your hands back to the ankle. Repeat 3-6 times.

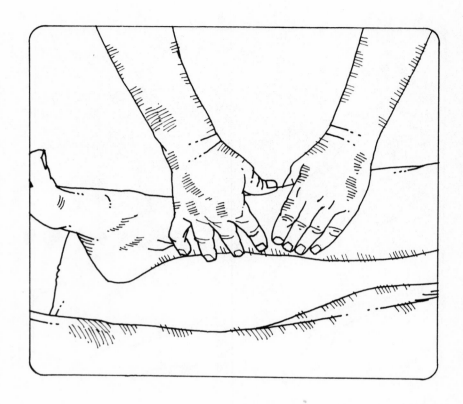

3. With one hand, grasp the leg just above the ankle. Use the thumb of your other hand to petrissage the muscle outside the shinbone from ankle to knee. The palm side of your fingers will maintain contact with the inner side of the shin but will be held flat rather than hooked. This will avoid irritating a large branch of the sciatic nerve that runs just behind the inner side of the shin bone. Move the grasping hand up the leg, ahead of the petrissaging hand. (Petrissage should be done within the crescent formed by the grasping hand and on the raised tissue.) Repeat 3-6 times.

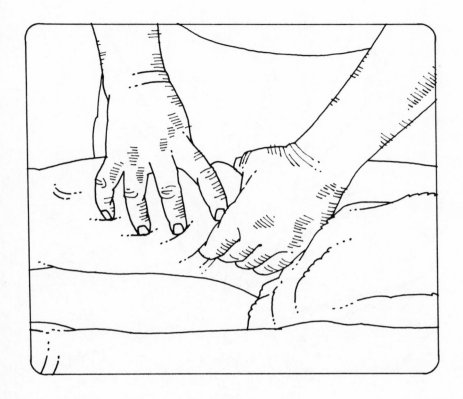

4. Continue to work upward from knee to thigh. But now use both your thumb *and* fingers to petrissage. (On a large or fleshy thigh, work in two to four inch sections up from knee to thigh until you have massaged the entire area.) Repeat 3-6 times.

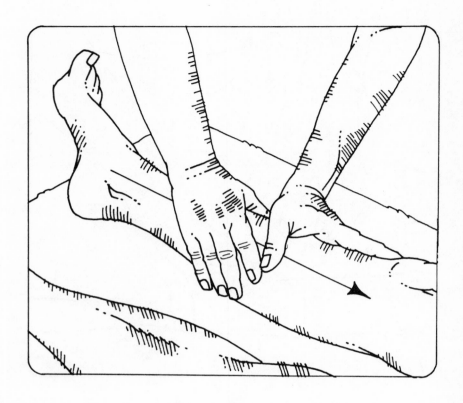

5. Effleurage the leg from ankle to upper thigh 3-6 times. Slide your hand across the kneecap so that you maintain skin contact, but avoid bouncing onto the thigh.

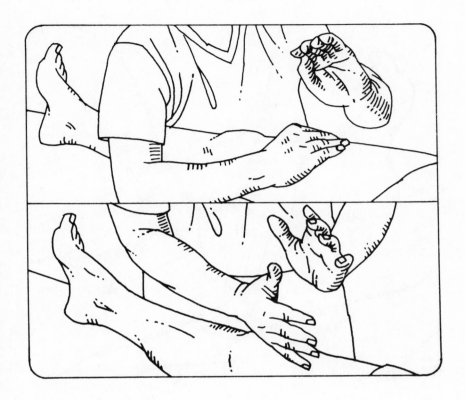

6. (Optional because some people do not care for it.)
Hack (2-3 times) and cup (2-3 times) back and forth from
ankle to upper thigh.

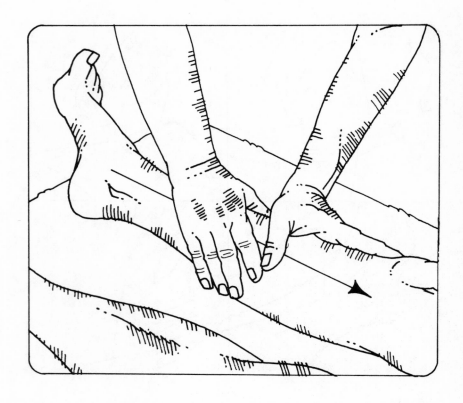

7. (Include this step *only* if you hack and cup.) Effleurage from ankle to upper thigh 3-6 times.

8. Move to the other side of the person and repeat the steps on the other leg.

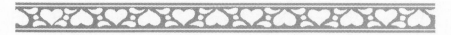

The Abdomen

Abdominal massage must be done on the bare skin because it is ineffective through clothing. It is especially helpful in reducing stress and tension that affect the abdominal area. This massage is also of particular benefit for those who suffer from irregularity. See Massage to Improve Regularity on page 84.

Precaution
Do not massage the abdomen if there is any sharp or pulsating pain, particularly in the lower right side. (Massaging during pregnancy requires special care. See Pregnancy Massage on page 91.)

Position
The person to be massaged will lie face up on a firm bed or other massage surface. For comfort, place a small pillow beneath the head and a bolster beneath the knees. You should be to the right of the person.

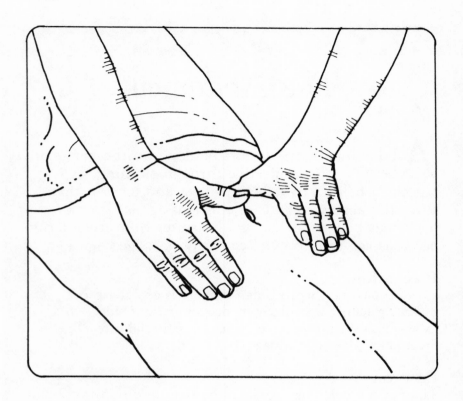

Sequence

1. Spread oil over the abdomen with light random strokes such as you would use to apply suntan lotion.

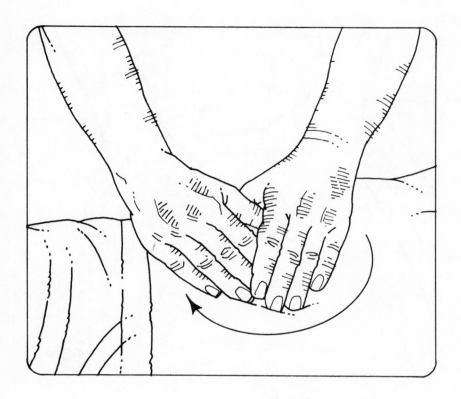

2. Overlap the fingers to form a small Christmas tree with the hands. Use the palms and fingers of both hands in a *clockwise* circular effleurage. This stroke *must always* be down on the left side of the abdomen to match peristaltic action. Massage in slow *gentle* strokes from below the ribs to just above the pubic bone area. Repeat 3-6 times.

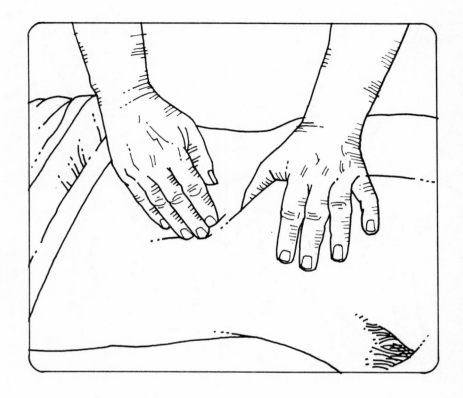

3. Place the palm of one hand flat against the bottom of the ribs to protect them from being accidentally tickled by your massaging hand. Petrissage with the fingertips in a general clockwise motion around the abdominal area (always down on the person's left side). Ask the person to tell you if you should use more or less pressure. There should be no pain. Cover the entire area in ever smaller circles. (It's like working from the outer edge of a spiral in to the center.) You end at the navel. Repeat the spiraling petrissage 1-3 times.

4. Repeat Step #2 to complete the massage.

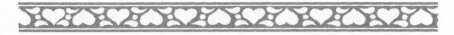

The Chest

Chest massage can be done through clothing, in which case you cover the clothing with a terrycloth towel (100% cotton) to protect your fingertips. Petrissage can be done through a towel, but effleurage can only be done effectively on bare skin.

Precautions
Do not massage the upper chest of anyone known to have any type of cancer. Noticeable dimpling or dents or a sunken or deformed nipple should be considered suspect enough to avoid massage. Do not diagnose *to* the person being massaged to avoid frightening or alarming the person. I usually suggest, very calmly, "The next time you see your doctor, have him or her check this condition." Discontinue massaging anyone who has any pain other than slight tenderness. Ask women if they are aware of any unusual breast conditions, and always use *extremely gentle* strokes on the female chest, particularly around a fibrocystic breast. (You may feel irregular, rounded masses in the breast.)

Position
The person to be massaged will lie face up on a firm bed or other massage surface. For comfort, place a small pillow under the head and a bolster beneath the knees. To begin, stand to the right of the person and reach across the chest to work on the side farthest from you. When you finish that side, move to the opposite side of the person and again work on the farthest side of the chest.

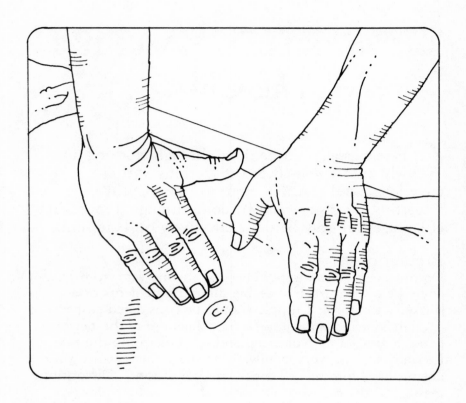

Sequence
1. Spread the oil with a gentle effleurage stroke.

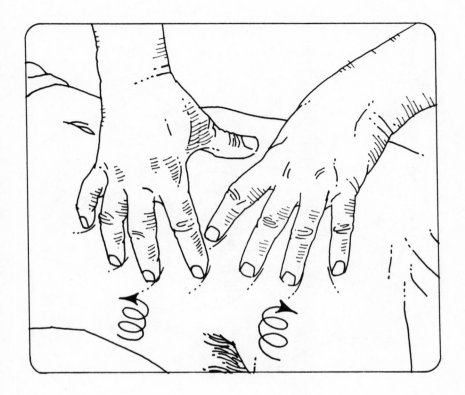

2. (For men.) Petrissage with the fingers of both hands *between* the ribs. Work inward toward the breastbone, following the curve of the ribs up from the side. Adjust the finger pressure as needed to avoid tickling the person. Repeat 1-3 times.

3. Switch to the opposite side and repeat Step #2.

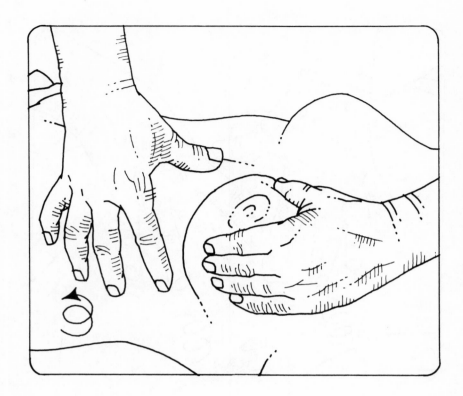

2. (For women.) Petrissage with the fingers of both hands *between* the ribs. Work inward toward the breastbone, following the curve of the ribs. *Do not* do the ribs directly beneath the breasts. Instead, cup the breast with one hand and with the other hand do a very gentle petrissage around the entire breast area where it attaches to the chest. (This is similar to the woman's monthly breast examination.) Repeat 1-3 times.

3. Switch to the opposite side and repeat Step #2.

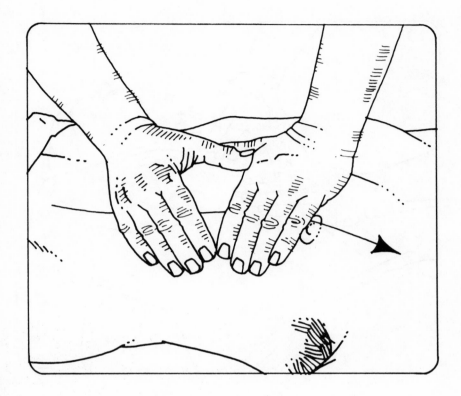

4. (For men.) Place your hands in the small Christmas tree position and do a *slow*, firm effleurage from the lower abdomen to the collar bone. Since you're working from the side of the person, you'll use a sweeping, sideways stroke. Use as many strokes as necessary to cover the entire area. Repeat 3-6 times.

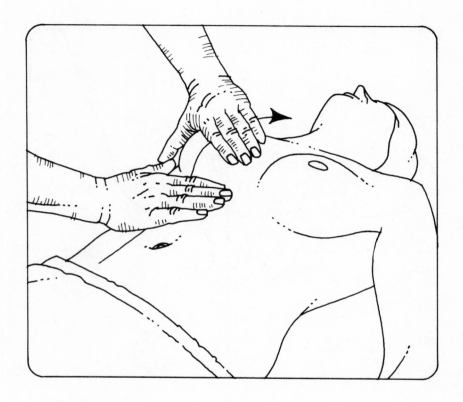

4. (For women.) Place your hands in the small Christmas tree position and do a *slow*, firm effleurage from the lower abdomen to the collar bone. Since you're working from the side of the person, you'll use a sweeping, sideways stroke. Cross up and over the breast area with *less* pressure than you would use on a man. Use as many strokes as necessary to cover the entire area. Repeat 3-6 times.

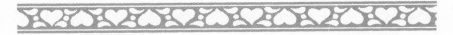

The Hands

Along with the face and the feet, the hands store an enormous amount of tension that can be removed by massage. The use of oils or hand creams is recommended, but you can do the massage without them.

The hand massage is very relaxing. When combined with a facial and neck massage it can contribute to restful sleep. This massage is a special gift you can give to anyone who is hospitalized or bedridden or in a nursing home. Do it slowly and be very careful when bending the person's wrist.

Precautions

Avoid massaging any injured portion of the hand or any area that is swollen or showing symptoms (redness, stiffness, swelling) of arthritis—especially knuckles or wrists. Hangnails can be aggravated by massage, so use care in massaging along the sides of the nails.

Position

This is a massage you can do while sitting side by side on a couch or across a small table. It is best done, however, with the person to be massaged lying down, face up on a firm bed or other massage surface.

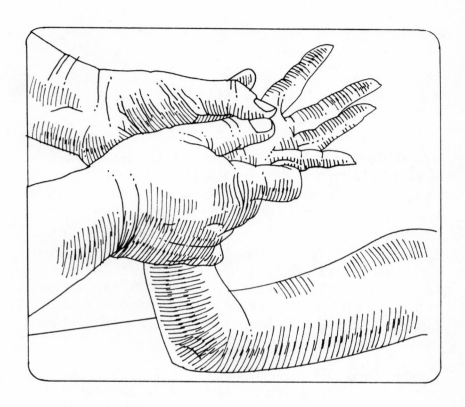

Sequence

1. If you are using an oil or cream, apply it with a gentle stroke. Rest the elbow and raise the forearm. The palm of the hand should face you. Place your thumbs in the palm and clasp your fingers around the back of the wrist. Use your thumbs to rock the hand backwards to the point of resistance, then release the pressure, letting the hand "bounce" back each time this point is reached. Do this 3-4 times. If the person reports any pain, use the point of pain rather than the point of resistance as the release point.

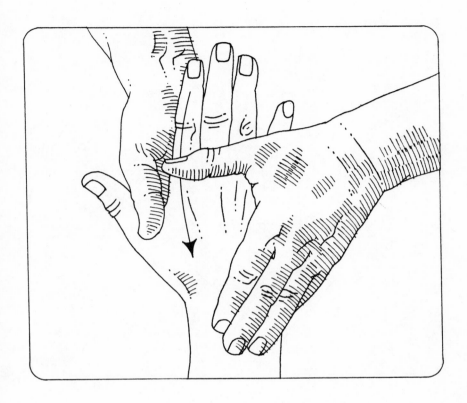

2. Hold the person's hand palmside down in one of your hands. Use the flat side of your thumb to gently effleurage the back of the hand. Stroke from fingertip to wrist, 2-3 times. Begin with the little finger side and work across to the thumb.

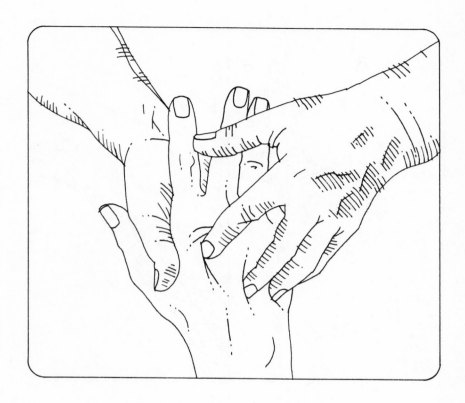

3. Continue holding the person's hand. You'll use your index fingertip to draw dime-size circles, but for this massage you *don't* lift your fingertip from the skin. You'll be "writing" a series of connected "O's," doing about 3 before sliding about 1/2" further and doing the "O's" again. Begin just behind the fingernail of the little finger and work all the way to the wrist. Massage *between* the bones of the hand from the base of the fingers to the wrist. Continue to do each finger (one at a time) and finally the thumb.

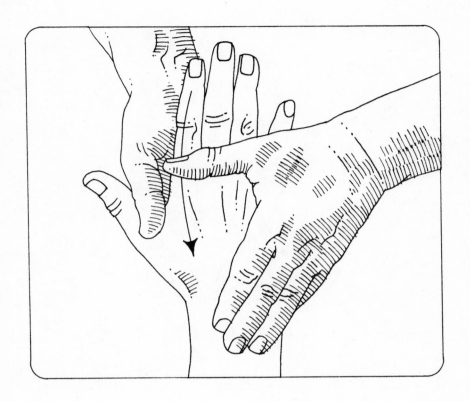

4. (Repeat of Step #2.) Hold the person's hand palmside down in one of your hands. Use the flat side of your thumb to gently effleurage the back of the hand. Stroke from fingertip to wrist, 2-3 times. Begin with the little finger side and work across to the thumb.

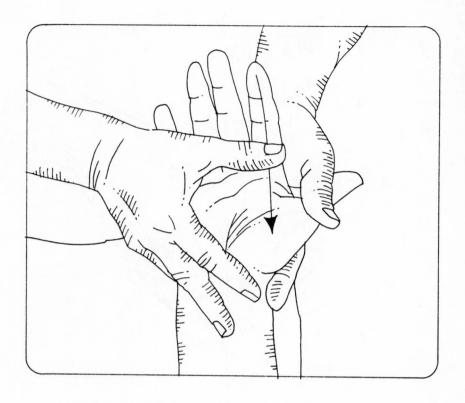

5. Hold the person's hand palmside up in one of your hands. Use the flat side of your thumb to gently effleurage along the palmside of the hand. Stroke from fingertip to wrist, 2-3 times. Begin with the little finger side and work across to the thumb.

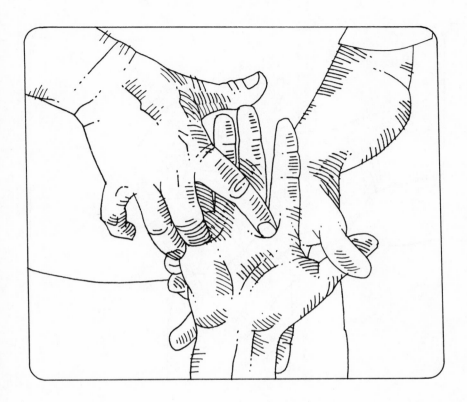

6. Continue holding the person's hand palmside up. Use your index fingertip to petrissage a series of connected "O's," doing about 3 before sliding about 1/2″ further and doing the "O's" again. Begin at the fingertip of the little finger and work all the way to the wrist. Massage *between* the bones of the hand from the base of the fingers to the wrist. Continue to do each finger (one at a time) and finally the thumb.

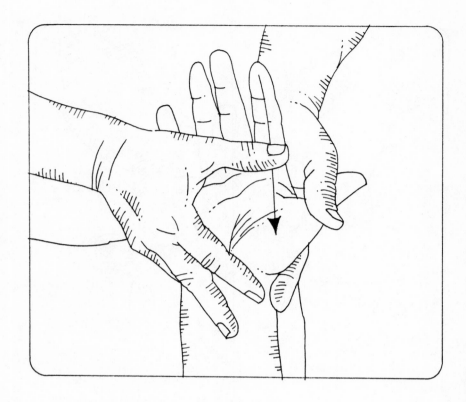

7. (Repeat of Step #5.) Hold the person's hand palmside up in one of your hands. Use the flat side of your thumb to gently effleurage along the palmside of the hand. Stroke from fingertip to wrist, 2-3 times. Begin with the little finger side and work across to the thumb.

8. Repeat the entire sequence for the other hand.

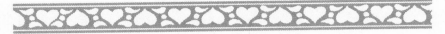

The Arms

The arm massage may be done directly on the skin or through a terrycloth towel, with or without oil. Persons with hairy arms should be massaged through a towel or with oil. (Working on the bare arm without oil pulls the hair and can be uncomfortable.)

This massage can be done for anyone and is especially helpful to those who have overused arm muscles at work or play. It is easy to do for yourself, but it is always more pleasant to receive.

Precautions

Do not massage closer than six inches from an arthritic wrist, elbow, or unhealed injury. Use of the circular fingertip massage (petrissage) and flowstroke massage (effleurage) toward the heart should stop six inches before an injury and should be restarted six inches past the injury.

Position

The person to be massaged can be seated beside you, but the preferred position is lying down, face up on a firm bed or other massage surface.

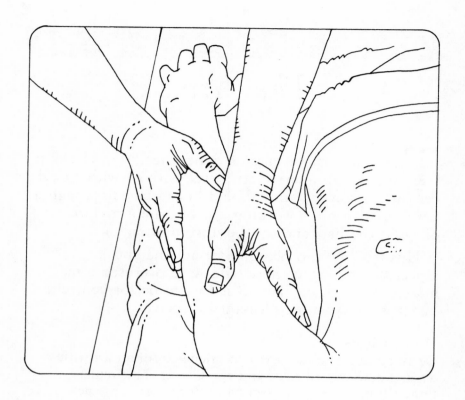

Sequence

If massaging through a towel, do only Step #3.

1. Spread oil over the entire arm with gentle effleurage.

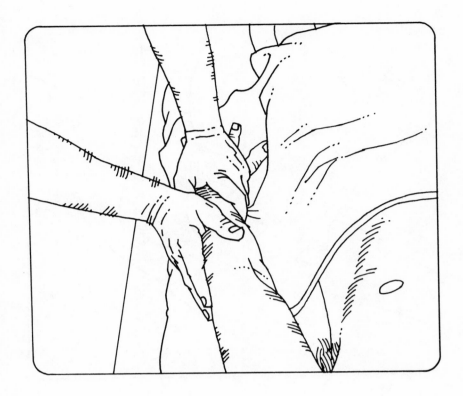

2. Hold the person's hand down to keep the arm straight and effleurage with your other hand. Make long, nonstop strokes from the wrist to the shoulder, 3-6 times. "Trail" your fingertips gently along the skin as you move back from the shoulder to the wrist. As always, forceful strokes are directed toward the heart.

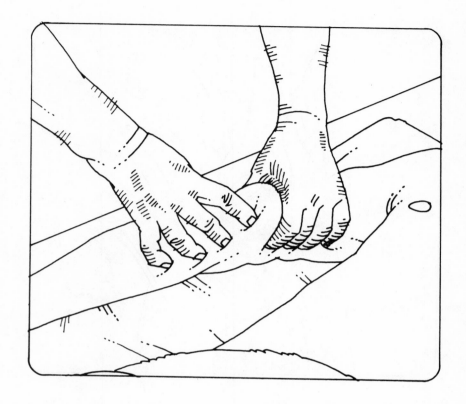

3. Gently pull the person's hand down to keep the arm straight. Use the thumb and fingers of your other hand to petrissage from wrist to shoulder, 3-6 times. (Use enough pressure to dent the skin, but you should cause no pain.) The hand not doing the petrissage will continuously grip and lift the arm tissue, always staying next to the massaging hand. The petrissage must be done on the raised portion of tissue.

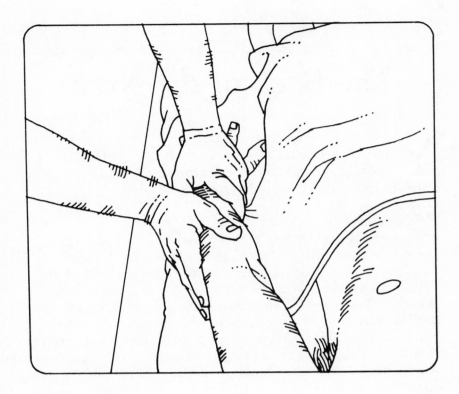

4. Hold the person's hand down to keep the arm straight and effleurage with your other hand. Make long, nonstop strokes from the wrist to the shoulder, 3-6 times. "Trail" your fingertips gently along the skin as you move back from the shoulder to the wrist.

5. Repeat the entire sequence for the other arm.

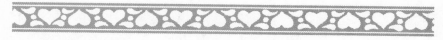

The Back of the Neck

Y ou can use a facial cream or an oil for this massage. Facial cream is better than oil if the skin appears dried or damaged by age or the sun.

Precautions

If the neck is sore or has been injured in any way within the past six months, the massage must be done lightly. (You can, however, do each motion for a longer period of time. The final effect is the same as that of a more firm massage.) There should be no twisting or stretching of the neck within six months of any injury. Motor and sensory nerves to the upper torso and arms come out of the cervical vertebrae of the neck. Twisting or stretching can aggravate any existing condition. Massage of the neck should be done with awareness of any problems and with great care.

Neck massage can often break the cycle of pain-cramp-pain, bringing relief from headaches and upper body fatigue. Some of the causes of neck pain include: sleeping without a pillow or in a draft, extended driving, or even sitting overly long at a typewriter or word processor.

Position

The person to be massaged should lie face up on a firm bed or other massage surface.

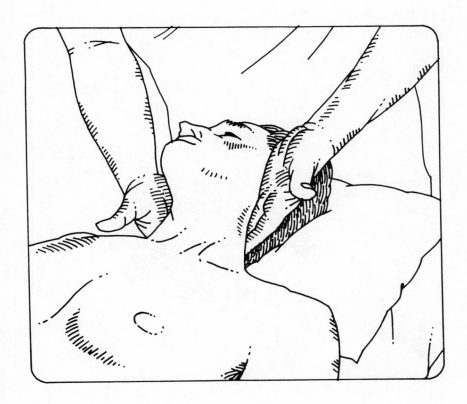

Sequence

1. Apply a small amount of cream or oil to the back of the neck using the flats of the fingers in a light but rapid circular stroke to warm the skin and stimulate circulation.

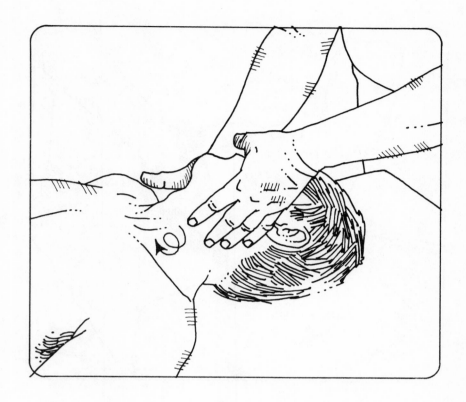

2. If you are able to massage with both hands at the same time, work on both sides of the neck simultaneously. Otherwise, do one side of the neck at a time. Petrissage up and down the neck from the base of the skull to the top of the shoulders. Repeat 8-10 times. The massage should be done firmly but without causing pain. Be sure to ask the person whether you are applying too little or too much pressure.

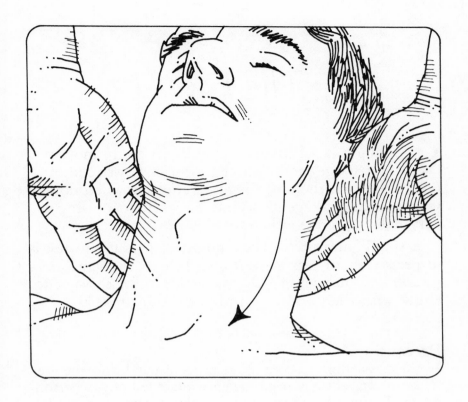

3. Effleurage, if neck is long enough, should be done with the flats of the fingers in firm strokes from the base of the skull downward into the upper back.

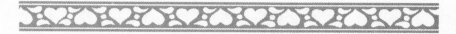

The Face

Giving a facial involves circular fingertip motion (petrissage) and a special form of flowstroke (effleurage). Although it is more effective when done with oil, the massage may be done without it, using a very light fingertip effleurage.

A simple measure of the amount of pressure to use is to press your fingers to your own face in the same areas you will be massaging. Of course you will also want to check with the person to find out if the stroke is comfortable.

Precautions
Avoid massaging the bony ridge immediately below the eye socket to prevent any injury from contact lenses. A person may well forget to tell you and you may forget to ask. Also, the skin below the eye socket is very thin and contains many fine blood vessels. Massage can bruise or break these blood vessels, causing—among other things—darkness under the eyes.

Position
When you're working on the full body, give this massage from above and behind while the person lies face up on a firm bed or other massage surface. Otherwise, have the person lean back in an overstuffed chair or a chair with a pillow draped over the back. The massage should not cause neck pain.

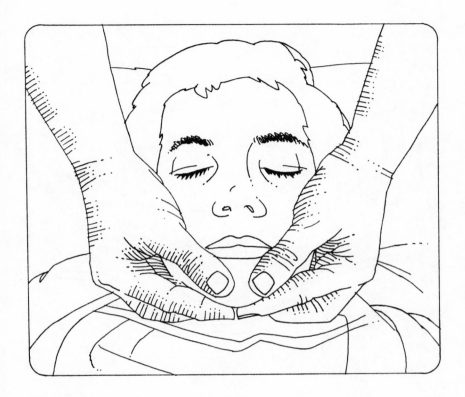

Sequence

1. Draw your fingertips lightly from the center of the chin to the base of the ears, just above the top of the lower jawbone. A major facial nerve ganglion (junction) is located here.

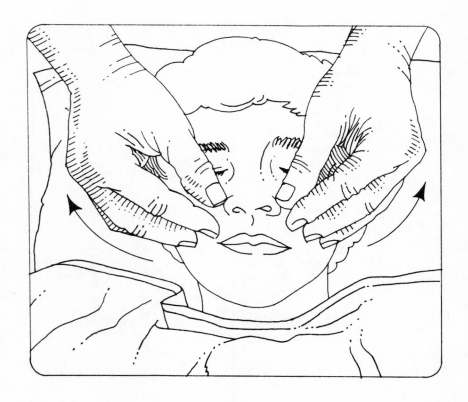

2. Continue drawing your fingers from the center of the face to that same point under the ears, moving up an inch at a time until you reach the hairline. (These motions soothe the skin and spread the oil if you're using it.) Be careful to avoid getting oil in the eyes.

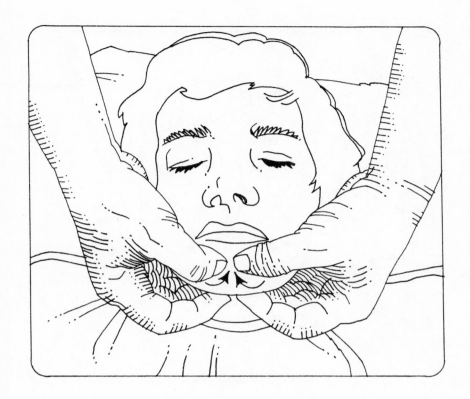

3. Petrissage with the first two fingers and thumbs of each hand. Begin at the center of the chin, at the base of the tooth roots above and below the edge of the lower jawbone. Massage under and along the inner edge of the lower jawbone, 2-5 times. Then lift your fingers slightly and move them about one-half inch closer to the ear and jaw juncture and repeat the petrissage. Continue this sequence until you reach the base of the ear. (Use enough pressure to move the skin against the bone. The fingers *should not* distort or pull the skin in such a manner as to cause it to stretch.)

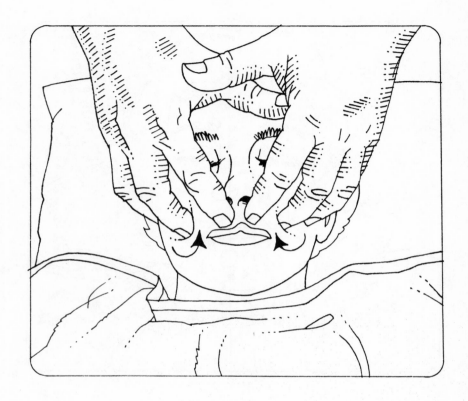

4. Now repeat the above massage sequence, but *begin* this time at the center of the upper lip. Follow the line that you can feel between the cheekbone and the roots of the upper teeth all the way to the base of the ear.

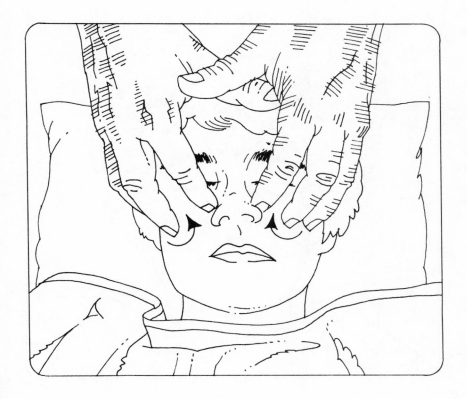

5. Place your *index fingertips only* on the cheekbones on both sides of the nose above the flare of the nostrils. You will feel the junction of the cheek bone with the curve of hard bone that forms the nose. Make the circular motion with your fingertips on this junction 2-5 times with firm pressure. (This area is often more tender than the rest of the face because it contains the ganglion of a major sinus nerve. Massage at this point will often relieve sinus congestion and headache.)

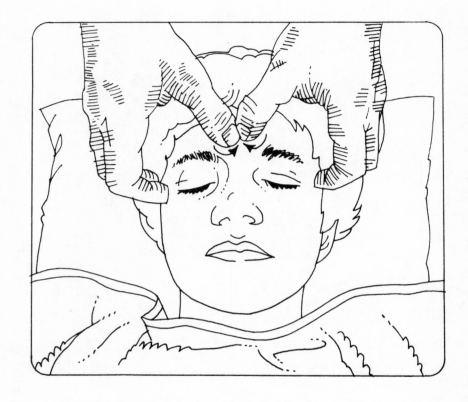

6. Place the first two fingers of each hand in the hollows of the temples and the thumbs at the bottom center of the forehead between the eyebrows. Petrissage with curled fingers and thumbs 2-5 times. Then keep your fingers in place at the temples, but move your thumbs up the forehead one-half inch. Repeat the massage 2-5 times. Continue moving your thumbs up one-half inch and massaging each time until you reach the hairline.

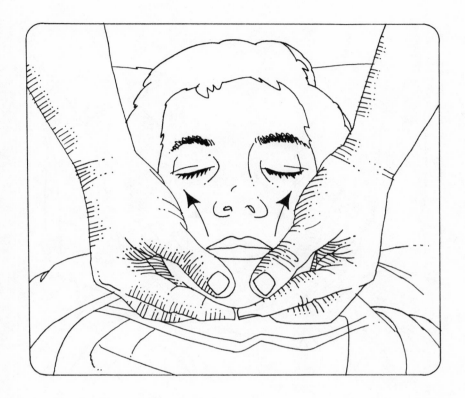

You're now ready to do the special flow stroke (effleurage) used in the facial massage.

A. Cup the lower jaw with both hands, with your thumbs and fingertips together at the chin.

Press the skin firmly inward against the facial bones for a moment.

Slowly release the pressure and draw your fingertips lightly back to the ears.

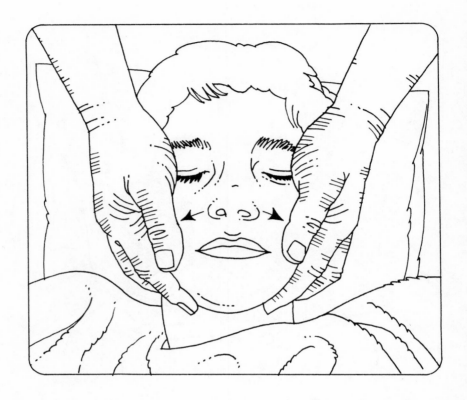

B. Cup the cheekbones with both hands, with your thumbs and fingertips at the sides of the nose.

Press the skin firmly inward against the facial bones for a moment.

Slowly release the pressure and draw your fingertips lightly back to the ears.

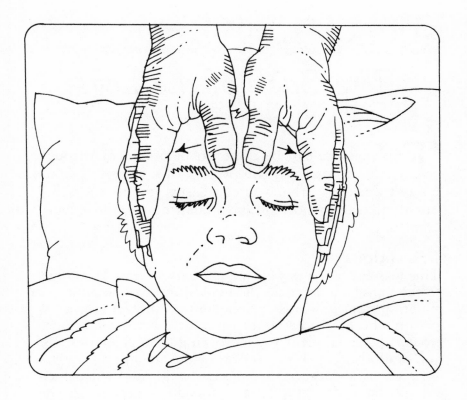

C. Cup the temples, with your thumbs touching along their full length at the center of the forehead.

Press the skin firmly against the forehead.

Release the pressure and slowly stroke the full length of your thumbs sideways over the forehead and down to the temples. Then use your thumbs to stroke the skin back from the temples to the ears.

Do the complete A-B-C sequence 2-3 times.

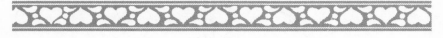

The Back of the Legs

This massage can be done on bare skin or through the clothing with the overlay of a terrycloth towel. It's not a massage that you can easily give to yourself, but there are portions of it you can do to relieve leg cramps.

Precautions
This massage involves working all the way from the ankle to the top of the buttock. It should not be done on anyone suffering from phlebitis or varicose vein problems or a person who has had a recent leg injury. Such conditions would not be visible if you're working through clothing, so you must check with the person before attempting any massage. Diabetics with leg ulcers should not be massaged even if the ulcers appear healed, as vein damage inside the leg, not evident to the eye, may still be occurring.

Position
The person to be massaged will lie face down on a firm bed or other massage surface, forehead and chin on a soft pillow. To relieve the natural tension of the muscles, place a bolster or a rolled pillow under the person's ankles. Work on the right leg from the right side and the left leg from the left side. Do not attempt to work *across* the person's legs because it will be hard on your back and prevent you from exerting the proper pressure.

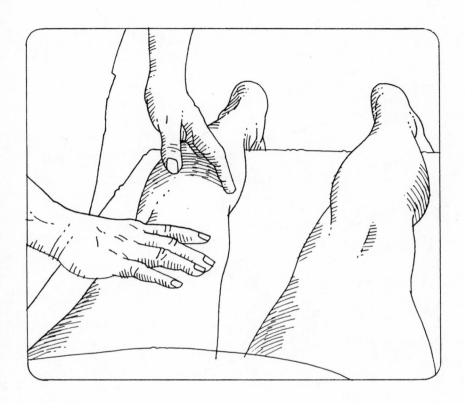

Sequence

If massaging through clothing, do only Steps #3, 4.

1. Spread oil over the entire leg with gentle effleurage.

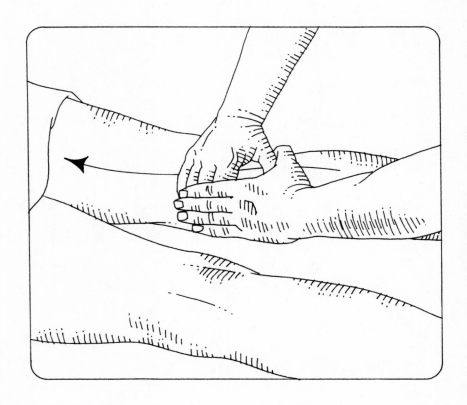

2. Overlap your hands in the small Christmas tree position. Do a heavy effleurage from the ankle all along the leg and release at the top of the buttock. Allow your fingertips to "trail" lightly along the skin as you move back to the ankle. Do 3-6 of these strokes.

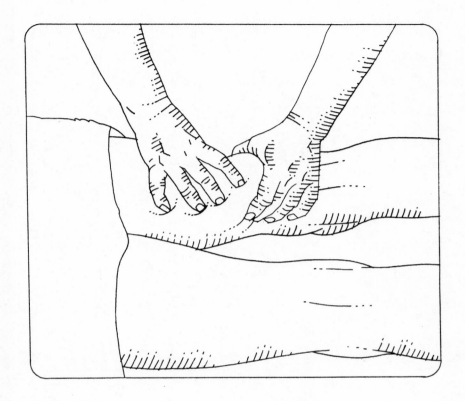

3. Begin petrissaging at the ankle. Grasp the area to be massaged with one hand. (Your thumb and index finger will form a "C.") Petrissage with the curled fingers and thumb of your other hand. Either the fingers or the thumb should be working within the "C." Perform each motion 3-6 times. Slide your hands up 1-2" and repeat. Continue all the way to the base of the buttock.

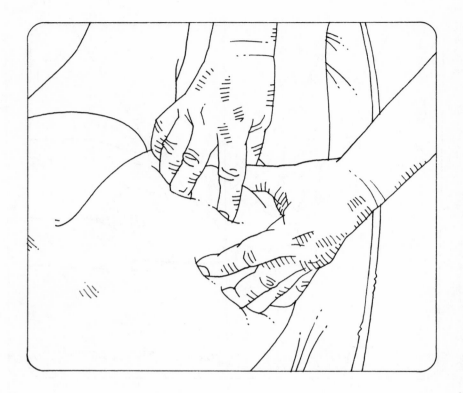

4. On the buttock, petrissage with the fingertips of both hands doing 6-10 dime-size circles at each position. Massage the center and outer edge of the buttock simultaneously, working from bottom to top. Slide your hands up about 1″ at a time and repeat the petrissage at each position. A fairly heavy pressure may be used on this large, dense muscle. Repeat about three times.

5. Repeat Steps #2, 3, 4 on the other leg.

This is an excellent massage for joggers and runners as well as those who spend a lot of time seated behind a desk or steering wheel. Sitting tends to decrease blood circulation to the legs and can cause leg problems, especially cramps and cold feet. The leg and sciatic nerve massage is effective in improving muscle tone.

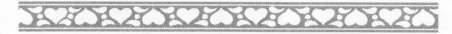

The Lower Back

Although you can do this massage through the clothes overlaid with a terrycloth towel, it is best done directly on the bare skin with warm oil. This is not a massage you can do for yourself. Learn how to combine the Lower Back Massage with the Upper Back and Shoulder Massage.

The cramping of back muscles and the resulting nerve blocks lead to many physical ailments that can be lessened or eliminated through regular use of back massage.

Precautions

Ask whether the person has had any recent injuries or suffers from back problems—such as a slipped disc—that could be affected by the massage. If so, a lighter but longer lasting massage is indicated if massage is to be permitted at all. Check the back yourself and don't massage anyone who has acne or any obvious swelling or inflammation. Petrissage should be done *between* or *alongside* any underlying ribs or spine rather than directly on them.

Position

The person to be massaged will lie face down on a firm bed or other massage surface, forehead and chin on a soft pillow. To relieve the natural tension of the muscles, place a bolster or a rolled pillow under the ankles. If you are right-handed, stand or kneel at the left side of the person; if you are left-handed, stand or kneel at the right side.

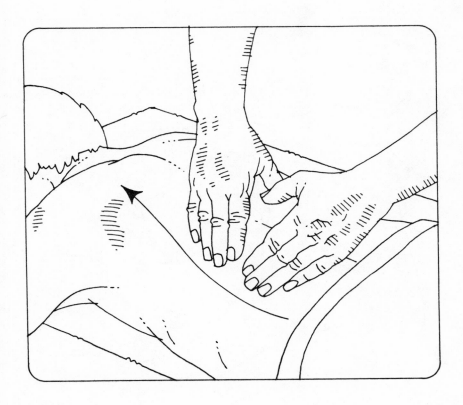

Sequence

If you're doing this massage through clothing, do Step #3 only.

1. Spread warm oil over the entire back, using gentle effleurage.

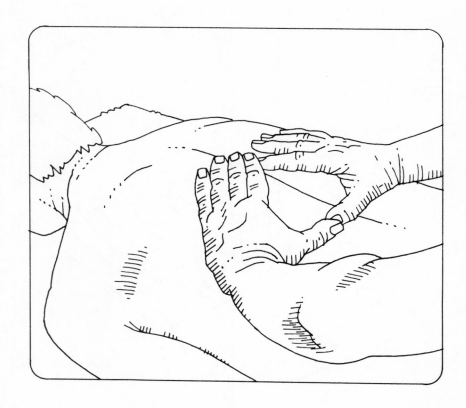

2. Form your hands in the large Christmas tree position. Do a heavy flowstroke from the waist to just over the top of the shoulders. Cover the entire back at least 3-6 times to soothe and warm the skin.

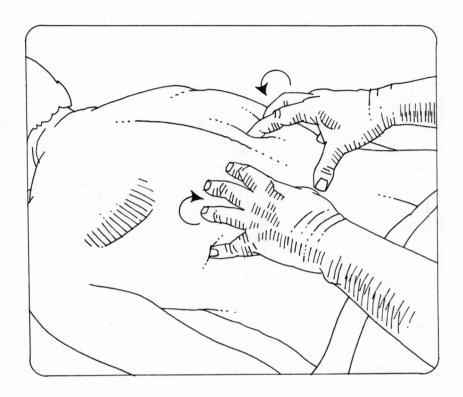

3. Use the fingertips and thumbs of both hands to petrissage the entire back 3-6 times, working from the waist to just over the top of the shoulders. Consider the back as a ladder. Begin at the bottom. Massage from the outer edges in toward the spine and then move your hands up 1-2″ to the next "rung."

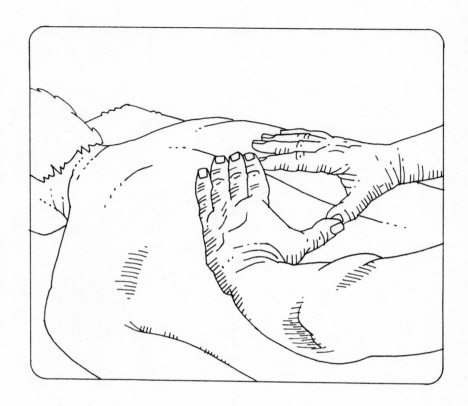

4. Form your hands in the large Christmas tree position. Do a heavy flowstroke from the waist to just over the top of the shoulders. Cover the entire back 3-6 times to soothe and warm the skin.

5. (Optional) If you want to give a more intensive massage, include the Deep Shoulder Blade Massage from page 78.

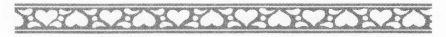

The Upper Back
and Shoulders

T his massage requires that you work on bare skin.
It's an excellent massage to give at the beach while
applying suntan lotion. In that case, the lotion is the
oil.

Precautions
Many people have injuries that aren't obvious to the eye.
Whenever working on the upper back, make sure to ask if
there have been any recent injuries such as whiplash.
Knowing the person's physical condition makes for a better
massage because you'll know how lightly or firmly to stroke.

Avoid massaging on the spine, and massage lightly wherever
you feel bone directly beneath the skin.

Position
The person to be massaged will lie face down on a firm bed
or other massage surface, forehead and chin on a soft
pillow. If you are right handed, your right forearm will be
across the person's back.

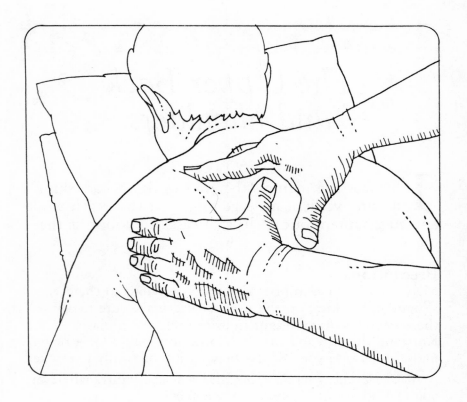

Sequence

1. Apply oil with light, random strokes such as you would use to apply suntan lotion.

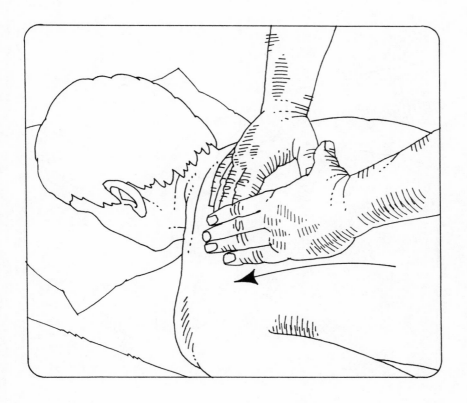

2. Overlap the fingers to form the small Christmas tree
with the hands. (This enables you to apply an even,
powerful stroke.) Effleurage with the palms of both hands.
Massage in rapid, forceful strokes from below the shoulder
blades, upwards to the neck, 3-6 times.

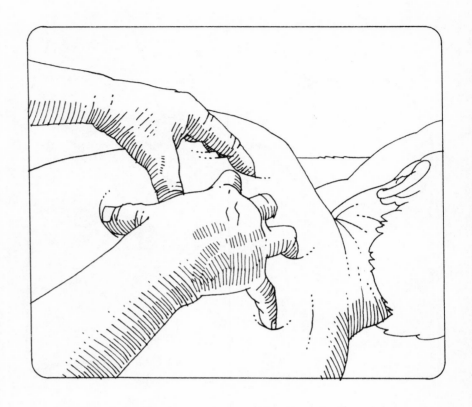

3. Petrissage with fingers and thumbs in the curled position. Draw dime-size circles on the skin, beginning at the lower and outer edge of the shoulder blades, 3-6 times. Lift your fingers, but maintain light skin contact, and replace them about 1″ closer to the spine. Repeat the petrissage.

Imagine the back as a ladder. Massage from the outer edges toward the center of each rung. Then move up a rung (about 1-2″) and massage again from the outer edge toward the center. Continue until you reach the tops of the shoulders.

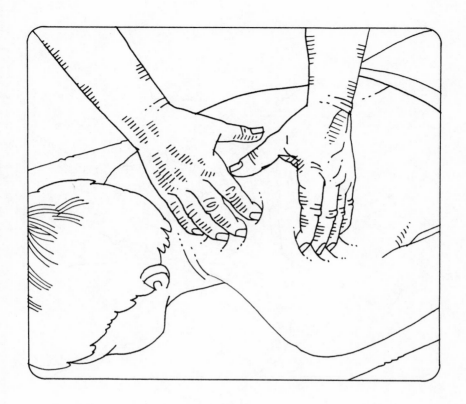

4. Petrissage the large muscle atop the shoulder all the way to where it joins the neck, 3-6 times.

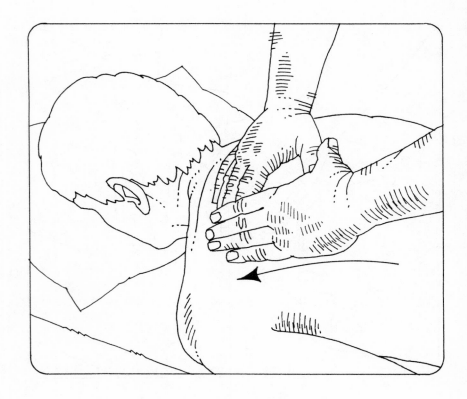

5. (Repeat of Step #2.) Overlap the fingers to form the small Christmas tree. Effleurage with the palms of both hands. Massage in rapid, forceful strokes from below the shoulder blades, upwards to the neck, 3-6 times. This completes the sequence, but you may repeat the entire sequence as necessary, to remove any remaining tension or stiffness.

Hand and Finger Fatigue
If you find using the fingertips of one or both hands too fatiguing, petrissage with overlapping fingers. See page 37. Perform the petrissage with the tip of the second finger only. Be very careful in using this technique because your fingertip can exert intense, hurtful pressure.

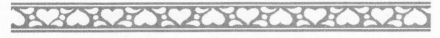

The Deep Shoulder Blade

This is a specialty massage that anyone will enjoy, but it is designed for people who lack shoulder mobility or suffer from bursitis. It is a method for massaging *behind* the shoulder blade and is an excellent follow-up to the Upper Back and Shoulders Massage.

Precautions
The position for this massage with the arm bent across the back is a difficult one for some people to get into, so you may have to help. *Move the person's arm slowly and carefully.* Any sudden motion can cause pain.

Position
The person to be massaged lies face down on a firm bed or other massage surface with forehead and chin on a soft pillow and places one arm straight down at the side.

Very slowly, bend the arm inward at the elbow so that the hand points at, or lies over, the small of the back. The desired elevation of the shoulder blade is that point where, if you press down on it with the palm, the blade will move down and "bounce" back freely. It will feel like compressing and releasing a soft rubber ball. Adjusting the arm and hand position on the back may be necessary to achieve this result because in some positions, the shoulder blade will be raised but will not easily compress.

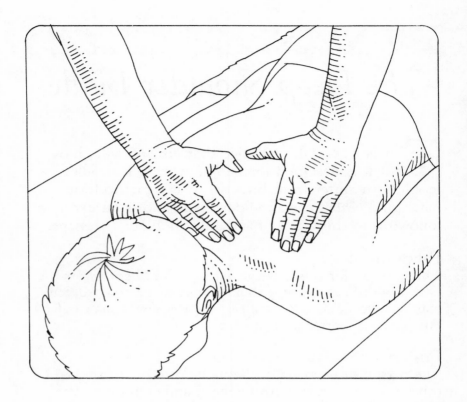

Sequence

1. Apply oil to the shoulder blade area with light, random effleurage.

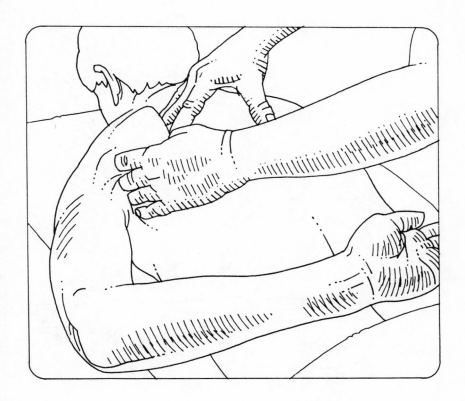

2. Petrissage with your fingertips on the raised tissue that
stretches from the edge of the shoulder blade to the back.
Move around the area, petrissaging 3-6 times in each spot.
(For people with shoulder problems, this will require at least
three minutes of petrissage for each shoulder blade.)

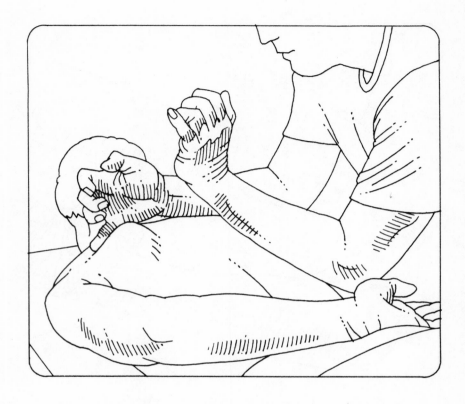

3. When the tissue feels warmer and more pliable due to an increased blood supply to the area, you are ready to use the soft heel of your hand to do the German hammer. *Gently* and *rapidly*, strike downward (with the fleshy part of your palm) around the raised edges of the shoulder blade about ten times. This will compress and release the tissue under the shoulder blade, pumping in fresh blood from the underlying arteries.

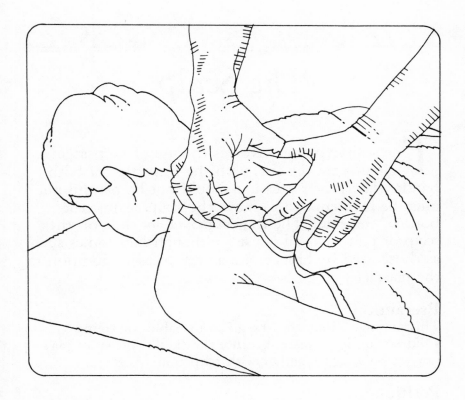

4. The final step involves kneading the muscle tissue gently through a towel. Use both hands to squeeze and release the tissue as though kneading a large lump of clay. Squeeze and knead slowly with the flat surface of the fingers and thumbs, holding them *straight* rather than curled. The objective is to knead, not grab or pinch. Firm but gentle is the rule.

Knead all the muscles around the shoulder blade, especially those atop the shoulder and near the spine. (The arm should be placed back at the side for this.)

5. Repeat Steps #1-4 on the other shoulder blade.

This massage can be repeated as needed to relieve upper shoulder pain or stiffness. Chronic shoulder pain that does not respond to massage should be referred to a medical doctor.

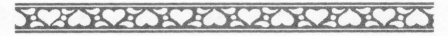

The Scalp

The scalp massage involves the use of petrissage (circular movement) with the fingertips of both hands. The finger pressure should not be painful but must be firm enough to move the scalp against the bone of the skull. The fingers *should not* slide on the scalp or hair. No oil is used, although hair tonics such as those used by barbers are a very pleasant addition to the massage.

Precaution
This massage should not be given to babies or young children (under 5 years) because the skull's soft spots may not yet be grown together with hard bone.

Position
The scalp massage is best done from above and behind. Have the person lean back in a comfortable, overstuffed chair or a chair with a pillow draped over the back.

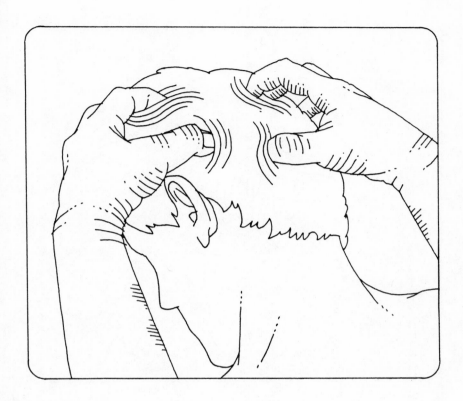

Sequence

1. (Use both hands.) Place your curled fingertips at the hairline of the forehead. Spread your fingers about an inch apart to cover the hairline from side to side. Petrissage with both hands, keeping your fingers *firmly* in place, moving the scalp against the bone. Rotate 5-10 times.

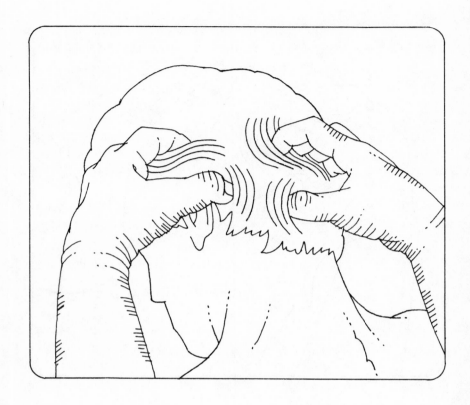

2. Move your hands back an inch and repeat the petrissage again 5-10 times. As you approach the nape of the neck, bring your fingers closer together so they will all remain within the hairline. Remember to keep your fingers and thumbs slightly curled to prevent hand fatigue.

This is an excellent massage for those who are bald. Simply follow the former hairline with all the same motions.

There is a plate of muscular tissue on top of the skull, somewhat larger and thicker in men than in women. As we grow older, this tissue tends to harden. Blood vessels carrying nutrients to the hair roots are constricted, resulting in hair loss or pattern baldness. (If you feel the scalp of a bald person, you will notice how little "give" there is.) Done regularly, this massage will soften the muscular plate, allowing increased blood flow to the hair roots.

In Swedish scalp massage the fingertips *do not* slide across the scalp. The proper technique avoids damage to existing hair and is often reported to encourage hair growth.

Scalp massage is extremely pleasing. It both relaxes and invigorates, and in many cases will remove the tension in the muscles underlying the scalp. It is this tension that causes certain types of headaches. One of the nicest things about this massage is that you can give it to yourself. Many people make it a part of their daily grooming routine. Scalp massage is also a great relaxer at any time and as a day-ender it can help bring on sleep.

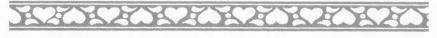

Wake Up Massage

This is a massage with benefits that last for approximately an hour, benefits that are most useful to anyone who is sleepy but must stay awake just a little longer. For example, the massage is used especially by students who need an extra hour of cramming for a test and drivers who are very near their destination but fearful of falling asleep at the wheel. It will usually provide a bit of extra—but temporary—alertness.

The massage is done on bare skin and without oil.

Precaution
If you are driving and want to try this massage, use it only if you have less than an hour's drive remaining. You may become exceedingly tired about an hour after using this technique.

Position
Sit comfortably. If you are driving, pull off the road and stop.

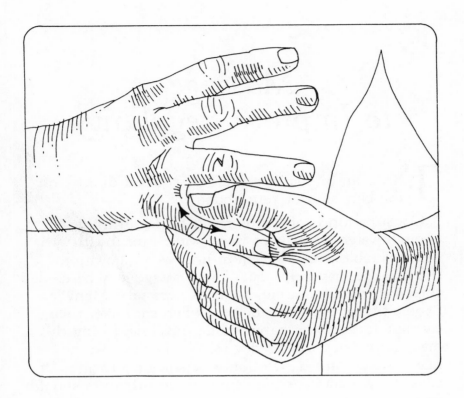

Sequence

1. Use the flat pad of your thumb (not the tip) to rub rapidly back and forth on the inner surface of the little finger of your other hand. Rub from the base of the finger to the first knuckle. Rub until the skin feels warm. Then do the little finger on the other hand.

2. Relax. Breathe slowly and evenly for about three minutes. After that, you may be more alert and awake, and this will last for approximately an hour. You can only make use of this technique once between sleep periods.

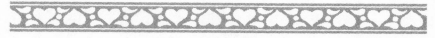

Massage
to Improve Regularity

This is an oil massage you give yourself directly on the bare skin of your abdomen.

Constipation is often the result of not drinking enough water. A glass of warm water mixed with two or three tablespoons of lemon juice as a followup to the massage may help you. This massage may be used three or even more times a day as necessary. Many people find it especially helpful when they alter their eating and drinking habits while traveling. Doing this massage once or more a day for two to three weeks may have a marked effect on a person's regularity. Of course, any persistent problem with constipation should be brought to your doctor's attention.

Precaution
Do not use this massage technique if there is persistent or pulse-like pain in the lower right abdomen. If there is intestinal gas present, the massage should be done *extremely gently*. The massage must be done only in a circular, clockwise direction (up on your right side, across the top to your left, down on your left side, etc.). Stop the massage immediately if you feel any sudden, sharp pain.

Position
Lie down on your back on any comfortable surface and place a large pillow beneath your knees. The knees should be raised to release the normal muscle tension of the abdomen.

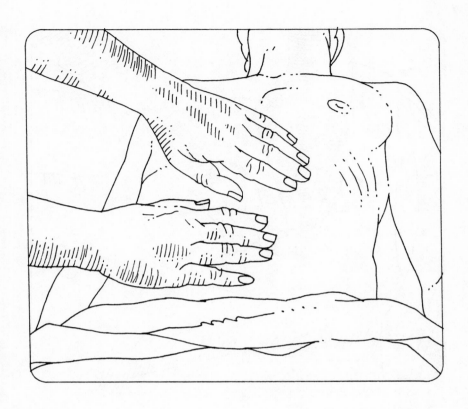

Sequence
1. Gently spread warm oil over the abdomen.

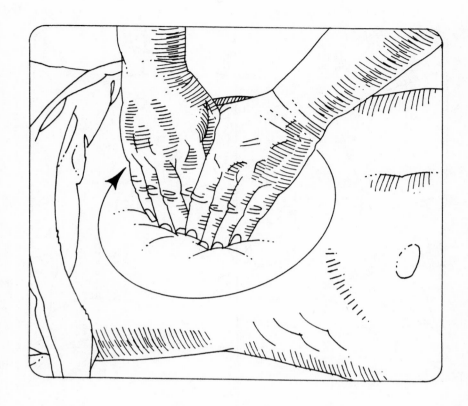

2. Hold your massaging hand flat with the palm to the abdomen. Make a clockwise flowstroke around the entire abdomen below the ribs and above the pelvic bone. (Main skin contact is with the palm, not the fingers.) Use a slight, steady pressure. Continue the circling motion about 15 times, or until the skin becomes slightly warm from friction.

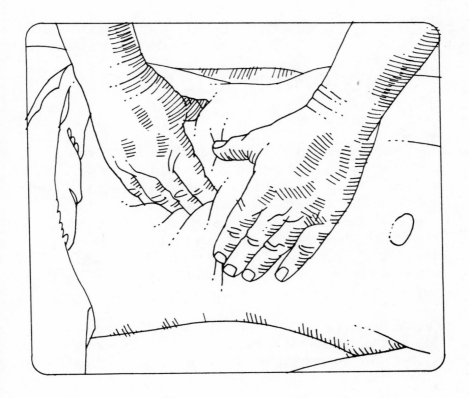

3. Use the fingertips only of your massaging hand to petrissage dime-size circles on the skin. Follow the same clockwise path as you did with the flowstroke. Use enough pressure to dent the underlying muscle tissue but not to the point of pain.

4. Repeat Step #2. Then use a towel to wipe off excess oil to avoid staining your clothes.

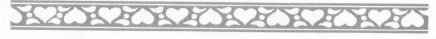

Morning Massage

Y ou can get off to a better start in the morning with a simple exercise and massage for sore shoulders. This is a procedure you do yourself without any oil. Doing this massage faithfully each day for as little as three weeks will stretch the shoulder muscles, improve the blood circulation, and lessen if not eliminate the problem. The day-by-day larger and larger circles that you're able to make without feeling pain will indicate how your muscle tone is improving.

Precaution
Do this massage immediately upon awaking, but don't continue it if you experience any sharp pain.

Position
Sit on the edge of the bed with your feet flat on the floor.

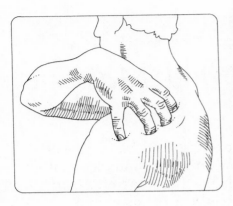

Sequence

1. Use the fingertips of your right hand to petrissage the top of your bare left shoulder, 10-20 times or until the skin feels slightly warm from friction. Repeat with your left hand on the right shoulder.

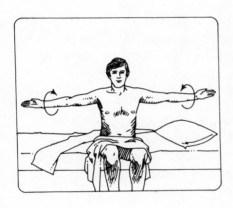

2. Extend both arms sideways from your shoulders, palms up. Move your arms in ten slow circles. Keep them straight and draw circles with your outstretched hands: forward, up, back, down, forward, etc. Complete each circle while counting *very slowly* to ten: "One-thousand-one, one-thousand-two. . . ." The slowness is crucial to the success of the exercise. Make each circle just large enough so that you feel some strain (just back from the point of pain).

3. After making the ten circles, repeat Step #1.

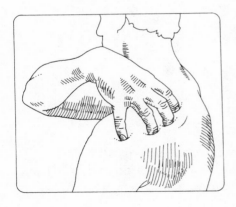

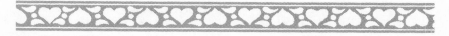

Eye Exercise and Massage

This self-administered exercise and massage will improve blood circulation in the muscles that focus and align the eyes. It has the most effect on people who are either nearsighted or farsighted.

Precaution
The place where you do the massage exercise should be well lighted and glare free. If possible, the illumination should be natural light.

Position
Sit at a desk or table and face a wall approximately 3-4′ away. Attach six playing cards to the wall with tape or tacks. Use cards number two through seven and arrange them in sequence in three rows. Leave one foot between each card and each row.

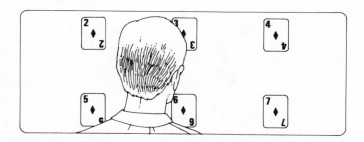

Sequence (to be done without wearing glasses)
1. Apply alternate warm and cool (not hot and cold) wet pack compresses gently over the eyes and temples. Make at least five applications each.

2. Use the fingertips of both hands to petrissage for 10-20 seconds in the soft, hollow part of your temples.

3. Blink both eyes *rapidly* as you count slowly to ten. Close your eyes and count slowly to ten. Repeat the blinking-closing sequence at least five times.

4. Review the pattern of the cards on the wall so that you can sense their positions with your eyes closed.

5. Begin slowly. Blink your eyes once and *instantly* focus on the top left number "2" of the first card. Blink again and *instantly* focus on the top left number "3" of the second card. Continue blinking and focusing only on the numbers until you have moved from two on through seven.

6. Repeat Step #5, blinking and focusing at a slightly faster pace.

7. Repeat Step #5, blinking and focusing at a still faster pace. Continue this over and over until you can't blink and focus any faster. Then stop and rest with your eyes closed for 1-2 minutes.

8. Keep repeating Steps #2-7 for a total time of at least ten minutes each day. End the treatment by repeating Step #1.

At the end of the first ten minutes of exercise and massage you will probably notice a surprising increase in your ability to see and even read without glasses. This ability will usually fade within a few minutes. But any muscle can be strengthened by regular exercise and you may be surprised by what will happen if you continue this exercise and massage daily over a period of at least three months. Although this technique is best done in the morning, many people won't have the time to do it then. Pick whatever time you're *most* likely to do it regularly.

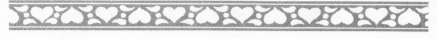

Relief for Leg Cramps

L eg cramps can be caused by everything from an
overweight abdomen pressing on a femoral artery
to nerve damage in the lower back or sciatic area of the
spine, from working in a seated position for too long a
time to a calcium deficiency in the bloodstream, from
rapid bone growth in children to excessive buildup of
lymph fluid in the legs of athletes.

Usually the best immediate relief can be obtained by
sitting in an alternate warm-cool bath and using both
hands to gently knead the leg muscles that are affected.
When the bath is not available, begin kneading just
above the ankle and work upward to the thigh.
Repeat, moving always up from the ankle to the thigh
until the cramping is alleviated. Doing the massage in
this instance may be done under a covering blanket or
towel to keep the skin warm.

Any cramping that persists should be referred to
your medical doctor. Leg cramps in the growth years
or in young athletes may indicate a vitamin or mineral
imbalance that a doctor can easily remedy.

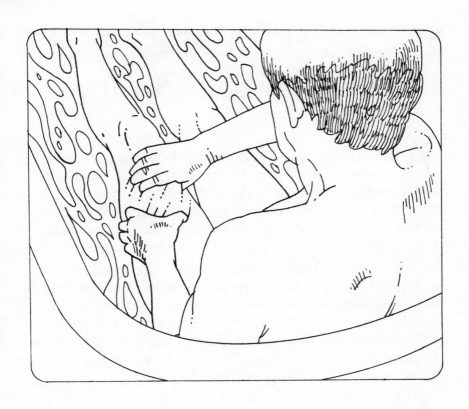

Relief for Joint Problems

Aches, pains, and swellings in the fingers, wrists, toes, and ankles are best relieved by 5-10 minute alternate soaks in cold and warm water, 1 minute of cold (not icy) to 10 seconds of comfortably warm (not hot) water. *Always* begin with the cold and end with the warm.

The joint should be exercised very slowly while immersed, but no motion is recommended if swelling is due to sprained or torn ligaments, as from a twisted ankle. The movement can be followed by a *gentle* kneading of the tissues, but don't work any closer than 3″ on either side of the painful joint. Keep the joint immersed while massaging.

Almost any joint pain can be relieved by using this cold-warm soak technique. After the soak and massage, dry the area carefully. If the painful area is in the legs or feet, lie down and elevate the leg on soft pillows so that it is slightly higher than the hip level. If the arm or hand is affected, sit and elevate the arm on a soft pillow so that it is about halfway to shoulder level. A good follow-up is to gently rub or dab on a fine skin oil, especially one containing aloe vera or lanolin.

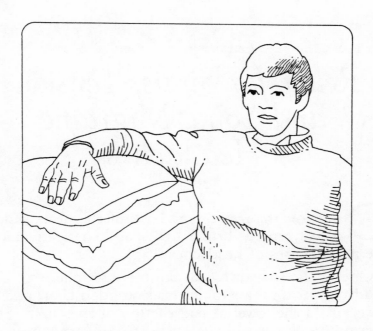

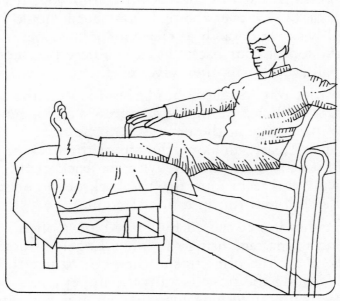

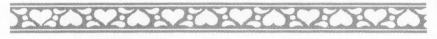

Relief for Sinus, Tension, and Some Migraine Headaches

Drafts on the face or the back of the neck, sudden or continuous bright lights, and stress are among the many causes of headaches.

One of the first things to do to try to relieve a headache requires a straight-back wooden chair and a towel. Fold the towel to pad the top of the chair. Sit in a position that will allow you to "roll" your neck from side to side over the pad. Your head should be leaned back far enough to create a "hollow" between it and the top of your back. Do a half-dozen or more slow rolls. This will often give relief.

Another way to relieve headaches involves the use of alternate cold and warm wet compresses and a gentle fingertip massage at the temples and the back of the neck, particularly all along the top of the neck in the bend formed by its juncture with the back of the skull. Following this technique, dry the back of the neck to avoid a chill and rub in a fine skin oil.

Sinus headaches caused by nerve blocks often respond to massage using the index fingers of both hands. Place the fingertips at the point where the bone forming the nostrils joins the upper cheek bones. If there is no tenderness, massage may not have any

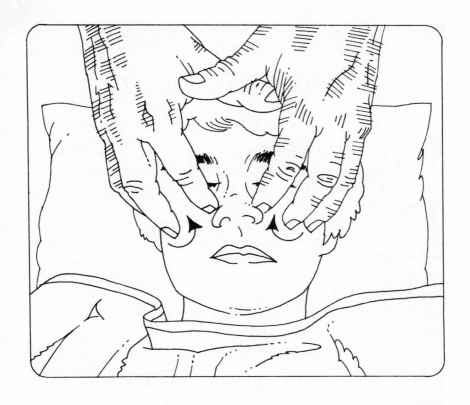

effect. (Tenderness is a possible indication that the sinus headache is of nerve origin.) If tenderness is felt, do a firm but gentle circular stroke (to the point of pain) for no longer than 30 seconds. Tenderness and the headache usually lessen or disappear during the massage.

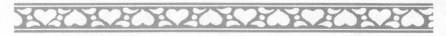

Pregnancy Massage

Massage during pregnancy helps to relieve stress and reduce back pain. The relaxation that results generally makes it easier for the woman to sleep. Although you follow almost the same routine in doing a full body massage on a pregnant woman as you do for anyone else, pregnancy requires some special care of the back and abdomen. You'll probably need extra pillows for support under the upper back and beneath the knees.

Precaution
Never do petrissage on the abdomen. You can do circular effleurage on the abdomen, but remember that it must be *very gentle* and always downward on the left side. The pregnant woman should feel no pain from your touch. Ask her to guide you in the gentle application of your hands. She will lie on her back and side but not on her stomach. Do not do any hacking or cupping.

Position (for the front of the body)
For the front of the body, the position is the same as for a woman who isn't pregnant, but give special attention to proper support with pillows, especially under the upper back and beneath the knees.

Sequence (for the front of the body)
Follow the regular front of the body massages except for the abdomen where you will do only *very light*, circular effleurage.

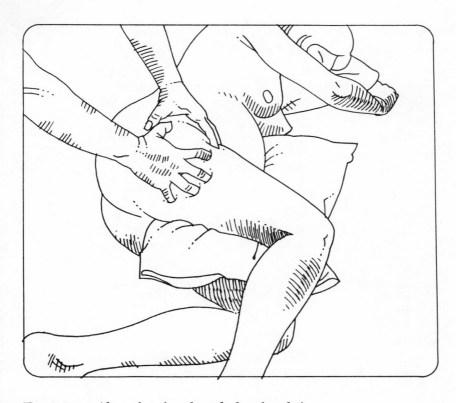

Position (for the back of the body)

The pregnant woman should lie comfortably on her side on
a firm bed or other massage surface. Place a pillow beneath
her head and support the abdomen with a second pillow.
Fit the end of the pillow slightly between the upper legs
and knees to prevent strain on the lower back and buttocks.

Sequence (for the back of the body)

1. Spread oil on the uppermost leg and uppermost part
of the back.

2. Effleurage and petrissage as you would a woman who
isn't pregnant, but petrissage much more gently on the
lower back and for a longer period of time.

3. When you finish one side, have the woman turn over
and do the other side of her back and legs.

Pregnancy Massage · **167**